the
NATURAL
FAT-LOSS
PHARMACY

Also by Harry Preuss

The Prostate Cure (with Brenda Adderly)
Maitake Magic (with Sensuke Konno)

Also by Bill Gottlieb

Alternative Cures
New Choices in Natural Healing
The Calcium Key (with Michael Zemel, PhD)
The DERMAdoctor Skinstruction Manual (with Audrey Kunin, MD)

Drug-Free Remedies to Help You
Safely Lose Weight, Shed Fat,
and *Feel Great*

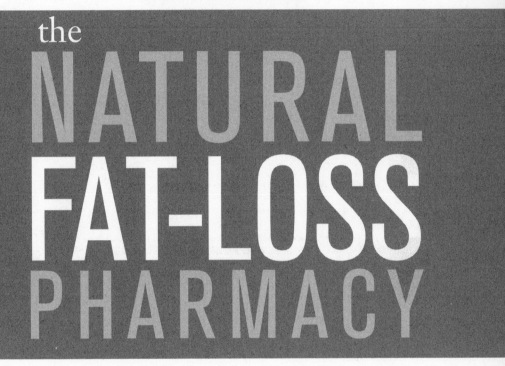

the
NATURAL
FAT-LOSS
PHARMACY

**HARRY PREUSS, MD, MACN, CNS
AND BILL GOTTLIEB**

RODALE

Notice

This book is intended as a reference volume only, not as a medical manual. The information given here is designed to help you make informed decisions about your health. It is not intended as a substitute for any treatment that may have been prescribed by your doctor. If you suspect that you have a medical problem, we urge you to seek competent medical help.

Mention of specific companies, organizations, or authorities in this book does not imply endorsement by the author or publisher, nor does mention of specific companies, organizations, or authorities imply that they endorse this book, its author, or the publisher.

Internet addresses and telephone numbers given in this book were accurate at the time it went to press.

Printed in the United States of America

Rodale Inc. makes every effort to use acid-free ♾, recycled paper ♲.

Book design by Mauna Eichner, Lee Fukui, and Susan Eugster

Rodale Inc. direct mail edition is published in 2007 under license from
The Doubleday Broadway Publishing Group, a division of Random House, Inc., New York

Library of Congress Cataloging-in-Publication Data

Preuss, Harry G.
    The natural fat loss pharmacy : drug-free remedies to help you safely lose weight, shed fat, and feel great / Harry Preuss and Bill Gottlieb.
        p.   cm.
    Includes index.
    ISBN-13 978-1-59486-706-4   hardcover
    ISBN-10 1-59486-706-2   hardcover
    1. Weight loss.   2. Dietary supplements.   3. Weight loss preparations.   4. Appetite depressants.   I. Gottlieb, Bill.   II. Title.
RM332.3.P74   2007b
613.2'5—dc22   2007020678

2 4 6 8 10 9 7 5 3 1   direct mail hardcover

RODALE
LIVE YOUR WHOLE LIFE™

We inspire and enable people to improve their lives and the world around them
For more of our products visit **rodalestore.com** or call 800-848-4735

To my wife, Bonnie,
and to my children—Mary Beth, Jeffrey, Christopher, and Michael
Harry

To Jan and Moshe,
who always turn my books face out
Bill

Contents

Acknowledgments

We'd like to express our gratitude to the many people who helped us in the creation of *The Natural Fat-Loss Pharmacy*. Thanks to:

Chris Tomasino, our agent, who helped shape the proposal and found a home for the book.

Leigh Erin Connealy, MD, and Tami L. Born, OD, for sharing their insights and experiences about the clinical use of natural supplements for weight loss.

Tracy Gensler, for working with us to create the Natural Fat-Loss Pharmacy Meal Plan.

Denise Getz, for her assistance in creating the Resource Guide of the book.

Lauren Hidden, the "virtual assistant," for her efficient and friendly help.

Marya Dalrymple, for shepherding the book at Rodale.

The many health, academic, and industry professionals who generously gave of their valuable expertise and time during the writing of the book, including: Richard Anderson, PhD; Debasis Bagchi, PhD; Joan Salge Balke, MS, RD; Dr. Doris Bell; Sarah Clark; Dallas Clouatre, PhD; Mike Danielson; Del Dorscheid, MD; Mary Enig, PhD; Dr. Jean-Michael Gaullier;

Dr. Michael Gonzales; John Grey, PhD; Julia Griggs Havey; Brenna Hill; James Hill, PhD; Elizabeth Jones, CCN; Peter J. H. Jones, PhD; Gilbert Kaats, PhD; Susan Luke, RD; Dr. Jit Maheshvari; Noboru Matsuo; Tom McCartney; Mary Jane Medlock; Jason Mitchell; Michael Murray, ND; Steve L. Nissen, PhD; Jeffrey Novick, MS, RD; Jason Odom; Sunny E. Ohia, PhD; Marlen Otten; Michael Pariza, PhD; Sanda Pecina; Pamela Peeke, MD, MPH; Christine Peggau; Heather Pena, MD; Nicholas Perricone, MD; Fred Pescatore, MD; Steve Pratt, MD; Caroline Richardson, MD; Julia Ross, MA; Dr. Filippo Rossi-Fanelli; Vicki Saunders, MS, RD; Kathryn Schmitz, PhD; Barry Sears, PhD; Mary Shomon; Joanne L. Slavin, PhD, RD; Linda Spangle, RN, MA; Sid Stohs, PhD; Marie-Pierre St-Onge, PhD; Bob Tennessen; Dixie Thompson, PhD; Dr. Ichiro Tokimitsu; Gretchen Vannice; and Dr. Margriet S. Westerterp.

Dr. Preuss would like to thank AdvoCare International, where he has served on the scientific-medical advisory board in the development of nutraceuticals, and the many other companies that have helped support his research at Georgetown University Medical Center into the efficacy of natural products for weight loss and for health: Interhealth Nutraceuticals, Maitake Products, Fuji Chemical, Pure Encapsulation, North American Herb and Spice, and Perricone Cosmaceuticals.

the
NATURAL
FAT-LOSS
PHARMACY

Introduction
Slimming Supplements:
Why Weight Loss Needs a Helping Hand

Let's cut to the chase—*your* chase, after a thinner, trimmer body. By putting into practice the information and ideas in *The Natural Fat-Loss Pharmacy*—by reading about and then deciding to take one or more of the weight-loss supplements featured in this book—it's likely that you'll be able to . . .

- Reduce fat absorption from your diet

- Burn more body fat

- Stop the formation of new fat cells

- Boost the power of exercise to burn fat

- Lose body fat when you diet, instead of calorie-burning muscle

- Build firming, toning muscle *while* you diet

- Curb your appetite at meals, eating less

- Feel less hungry between meals

- Mute your cravings for carbohydrates

- Stick with a reduced-calorie diet, instead of giving up

- Stop feeling depressed when you diet

- Get off a weight-loss "plateau," where pounds won't seem to budge

- Lose belly fat

- Lose extra weight

- Prevent weight regain after a successful diet

Yes, those are *some* of the possible benefits you can experience when you start taking one or more of the weight-loss supplements discussed in this book. (We say *some*, because that list of benefits, as big as it is, isn't comprehensive, and because many of these supplements can also help prevent and treat a wide range of health problems aside from overweight.) But before we tell you in more detail about these helpful supplements, let's take a moment to look at the scope of the weight problem—your problem, and America's problem.

ARE WE UNDER FAT ATTACK?

"Unless we do something about obesity," the surgeon general, Richard Carmona, told an audience at the University of South Carolina in 2006, "the magnitude of the dilemma will dwarf 9/11 or any other terrorist attempt."

Is our doctor-in-chief seriously saying that the real threat to Americans isn't Bin Ladin but being binge-laden? Isn't he exaggerating the impact of those extra pounds, trying to *scare* people into losing weight? Well, when you take a close look at the latest statistics on overweight from the government's Centers for Disease Control and Prevention, issued in 2006 . . . you can see why Dr. Carmona thinks knives and forks may be the real weapons of mass destruction.

To better understand those numbers, let's quickly review how scientists quantify overweight. To precisely define terms like *overweight, obesity,* and *extreme obesity*, they look at a person's body mass index, or BMI, an indicator of overweight and obesity based on a formula that divides weight by height. A person with a BMI of 25 to 29.9 is considered *overweight*; with a BMI of 30 to 39.9, *obese*; and with a BMI of over 40, *severely obese*. So, for example, a five-foot-five-inch woman is overweight at 150 pounds, obese at 180 pounds, and extremely obese at 240 pounds.

7 Out of 10 Ain't Good

The latest numbers show that 30 percent of Americans have a BMI under 25—that is, only three out of ten of us are *not* overweight! Which means, of course, that seven out of ten of us weigh too much. Among this large majority, 35 percent are overweight, 30 percent are obese, and 5 percent are extremely obese. Those percentages are higher than they were just a couple of years ago—and they've more than doubled in the past few decades! (In 1980, for example, about 15 percent of Americans were obese.)

But what's the bigger deal, anyway? So a lot of us weigh a little more than we used to. That's obviously not good, but is it really all that bad? Well, here's why fat is potentially terrifying. Those extra pounds aren't just unsightly. They're also unhealthy. Even deadly.

A Health Disaster

"A health disaster is happening," says Meir Stampfer, MD, professor and chairman of the departments of epidemiology and nutrition at Harvard Medical School, commenting on the government's new numbers. "Many health advances, like reductions in the rate of heart disease, are being obscured and diminished by the increase in overweight and obesity."

The metabolic mechanisms whereby extra pounds translate into extra disease aren't precisely understood. But statistics linking the two couldn't be clearer. And scarier.

Scientific studies show that people with a BMI of 25 or higher have an increased risk of:

- High blood pressure

- High cholesterol

- Heart disease

- Stroke

- Cancer (breast, colon, and prostate, among others)

- Type 2 diabetes

- Gallbladder disease

- Osteoarthritis

- Gout

- Sleep apnea and other respiratory problems

- Pregnancy complications

And although that list is long, and includes the major killers of Americans, it's also far from complete. Recent research, for example, shows that obese people have a lower pain threshold. (Overweight literally hurts you!) Another study shows that obese men are more likely to die in a car crash. (Who would have thought BMI could make a BMW less safe!) When you're overweight, it seems that *all* of your body takes a pounding.

How does our surgeon general suggest we deal with the threat of overweight? Should the government create a new agency—The Department of Fat—and begin issuing edicts against overeating? Put a surtax on doughnuts? Make fast food a felony? No, he says, each *individual* has to make "commonsense health decisions" that will help prevent weight gain and encourage weight loss.

And that's what *The Natural Fat-Loss Pharmacy* is all about. This book can help you make practical and positive decisions that will aid weight loss and maintenance. And if you're like most of us, you need all the help you can get.

BALANCED DIET AND REGULAR EXERCISE: ARE THEY ENOUGH?

You won't find us arguing about the two "commonsense health decisions" that are at the basis of effective weight loss. To shed pounds, you need to: (1) ingest fewer calories, and (2) burn more calories. In other words, you need to eat a little bit less and exercise a little bit more. Without that foundation, permanent weight loss is impossible—no matter how many supplements you take. Problem is, that foundation is getting harder and harder to build.

Huge Food

It doesn't take a tape measure, a food scale, and a PhD in mathematics to figure out what's happening to portion sizes in America: they're growing by heaps and mounds. For example, one study found that today's typical burger is about 3 ounces and 225 calories heftier than the average burger served in 1977.

But even though most Americans know that portions are more plentiful, and that eating everything that's put on your plate is a sure way to overeat . . . a survey conducted in 2006 shows that we don't practice much self-control—54 percent of those surveyed said they regularly cleaned their plate, no matter how much food they were served. That compares to 30 percent in a 2003 survey.

Between portions expanding at the speed of bite . . . and super-tasty foods like chips goading you to eat umpteen calories per commercial . . . and commercial after commercial enticing you to be oh-so-much-happier by buying New Food Fatty Treats . . . and mega-calorie convenience foods available 24/7, being told to cut calories doesn't quite cut it.

And advice to "exercise more" isn't much easier to follow.

Let's Not Get Physical

Between the remote and the mouse . . . the snow blower and the riding mower . . . and the drive-thru restaurant, the drive-thru pharmacy, and the drive-thru bank, we're not getting a lot of exercise. Government statistics say that only 23 percent of us exercise regularly, and 40 percent of us never exercise at all. We're a nation of couch potatoes. And we're being deep fried.

Facing the Facts

But you don't really need a barrage of facts and figures from the government to understand how difficult it is to cut calories and increase exercise. You know from personal experience. And if you've done the hard work of losing weight—if you've triumphed over fat—that victory was probably temporary: 95 percent of people who lose weight regain it.

Is there anything out there to make the daunting task of losing weight a little bit easier? Yes: the nutritional supplements and herbs featured in this book.

A LITTLE HELP FROM SOME FRIENDS

You'll read about many different kinds of weight-loss supplements in *The Natural Fat-Loss Pharmacy*. And each one can help you lose weight in a slightly different way. Let's look at them one by one. But remember, this is just an introduction—a brief summary. All the inspiring facts, and the scientific evidence to back them up, are in the rest of the book.

EGCG (green tea extract)—a safe way to boost metabolism. This herbal extract helps boost your metabolism *safely*, so that you burn more calories.

(By *safely*, we mean EGCG doesn't raise your heart rate and blood pressure, one of the possible side effects of ephedra.) For anybody trying to lose weight, increasing metabolic rate is crucial. Here's why . . .

Our bodies were genetically programmed thousands of years ago, when we survived by hunting and gathering. Whenever we could literally get our hands on nourishment, we ate as much as we could—and our bodies stored the extra calories as fat for times of nutritional scarcity. Well, say good-bye to the savannah and hello to the supermarket. We don't need to store fat anymore. But try telling that to your genes.

When you cut calories during a diet, your hunter-gatherer body "thinks" it's starving and automatically lowers your metabolism, to retain fat. That's why weight-loss diets are usually very effective in the first few weeks—and why after that initial success, the pounds shed oh so slowly.

EGCG can help your body burn many more calories per day, countering this natural impediment to weight loss. Plus, EGCG is a powerful antioxidant, protecting your cells from damage and thereby improving the health of your brain, heart, and immune, circulatory, and nervous systems. It may even help prevent cancer.

CLA (conjugated linoleic acid)—fat loss without dieting or exercise. A large-scale, two-year scientific study shows that you can lose 5 percent of your body fat and gain 2 percent more calorie-burning, body-trimming muscle—without diet or exercise—by taking this supplement for three months. Now that's what we call a helping hand. No, make that about twenty hands . . .

HCA (hydroxycitric acid, or Garcinia cambogia)—slowing down the manufacture of fat. This supplement works at the cellular level, reducing the formation of fat. In an eight-week study, people who took HCA lost four times as much weight as people taking a placebo, a fake look-alike pill. HCA can also reduce appetite (a crucial component of effective weight loss): in the same study, people taking HCA cut their calorie intake by 4 percent while those on the placebo increased their intake by 3 percent.

MCT (medium chain triglycerides)—a macho way to prevent weight gain. Several major scientific studies show that this unusual fat (found in coconut oil) can speed your metabolism, so you burn about 120 more calories a day. But the researchers who conducted the studies don't recommend MCT for weight *loss*. Rather, they say taking a supplement of the fat is a great way to prevent the slow but frustratingly sure weight *regain* that afflicts almost everybody who diets. And their results show that the supplement works particularly well in men—and seems to target their spare tires! Hey guys, admit it: if you could have a little help "changing" your spare tire, wouldn't you take it?

Chromium—balancing blood sugar. This trace mineral helps normalize blood sugar metabolism. And that's a big deal for weight loss. When blood sugar is stable, you're less hungry between meals and tend to eat less.

You also store less fat and make more calorie-burning muscle. In one study, overweight women on a diet who took chromium lost 84 percent fat and 16 percent muscle, while a placebo group lost 92 percent muscle and 8 percent fat.

Chromium can also help prevent (and even treat) type 2 diabetes, a devastating disease (common "complications" include blindness and kidney failure) that often afflicts the overweight.

Carbohydrate inhibitors—making a low-carb diet more fun. The tide has turned against low-carbohydrate diets: people have realized that it's more or less impossible to drastically reduce intake of one of the three macronutrients for a lifetime. (The other two are protein and fat.) But low-carb, high-protein diets can be a good short-term way to shed extra fat—and carbohydrate inhibitors make it a lot easier to go on such a diet, because you don't have to cut carbs quite as drastically. By taking either a starch- or sugar-blocker before a meal, you can have your cake (or at least a sensible slice) and eat it too.

Chitosan and other soluble fibers—foiling fat. These supplements can help block the absorption of fat. In one study, people given chitosan before a fatty meal absorbed 20 to 28 fewer grams of fat—180 to 250 calories! Taking a fiber supplement before a meal can also help you feel fuller faster, so you're less likely to overeat. And a fiber supplement slows down the absorption of the food you just ate, so your blood sugar stays balanced between meals, making it less likely you'll snack.

5-HTP (5-hydroxy-L-tryptophan)—cutting carbohydrate cravings. Scientific research shows that this amino acid dramatically reduces carbohydrate cravings—so much so that overweight women who typically overdid it on starches and sugars *effortlessly* reduced their caloric intake by as much as 1,000 calories a day, with more than 70 percent of those calories from carbs.

HMB (hydroxy methylbutyrate) and BCAA (branched-chain amino acids)—extra help for exercisers. These supplements protect and build muscle, a must for anyone using intense exercise as a way to help shed pounds or prevent weight regain. HMB has also been shown to prevent sarcopenia, the year-by-year, decade-by-decade loss of muscle mass that starts to afflict everybody around the age of thirty-five, and is a factor in the gradual and seemingly inevitable gain of weight around middle age (and around *your* middle!).

Savvy advice about the supplements we don't recommend. You'll also read about several weight-loss supplements that are widely advertised and used but that we don't recommend at the present time—either because there's not enough scientific evidence to support their efficacy, or because they might be unsafe.

Fortifying Your Intention

"The spirit is willing but the flesh is weak"—that well-known biblical saying definitely applies to the rigors of weight loss.

You're willing to lose weight. More than willing. But dozens of trials and temptations stand in your way, from an all-you-can-eat buffet to the zabaglione on the dessert tray. You need some effective assistance. The natural weight-loss supplements featured in this book can lend a helping hand. There's no reason not to reach out and take it.

A SAFER ALTERNATIVE TO DRUGS

Of course, you could also reach out for medication: a weight-loss drug like Meridia, which boosts metabolism, or Xenical (or its over-the-counter version, Alli), which blocks fat. Why not take a drug rather than a natural supplement?

Stated simply (and discussed at greater length in various chapters throughout this book): natural supplements, rightly used, are typically safer than drugs.

Meridia, for example, was linked to 124 hospitalizations for heart problems and forty-nine deaths.

Xenical has a range of unsavory side effects, including leaking oil from the anus, and explosive and uncontrollable diarrhea. Alli, the nonprescription version, may produce fewer problems, but may also be less effective. Of course, there are new weight-loss drugs headed for the market that are touted as an improvement on these drugs, like Accomplia. But how safe will they be? Safer than Vioxx? How does anybody know?

A Rogue's Gallery of Recalled Drugs

The problem with new drugs: even with the safety research conducted by pharmaceutical companies, nobody knows with any certainty the *long-term* safety of FDA-approved drugs. In fact, David Graham, MD, a reviewer in the Food and Drug Administration's Office of Drug Safety, testified at a congressional hearing that the FDA is "virtually incapable of protecting America" from unsafe drugs. Consider these examples that prove his point.

- Vioxx and Bextra—linked to thousands of deaths—were initially touted as safe and effective alternatives to nonsteroidal anti-inflammatory drugs like ibuprofen and aspirin.

- Baycol, a cholesterol-lowering statin, was withdrawn from the market after four years—and more than thirty deaths.

- Propulsid, a heartburn drug, was withdrawn after seven years—after killing more than one hundred people.

- Rezulin, a diabetes drug, was withdrawn after three years—and twenty-one deaths and one hundred hospitalizations.

The Seven-Year Rule

Those types of drug disasters are why the nonprofit Public Citizen's Health Research Group, at its Web site www.worstpills.org, recommends not taking any prescription drug until it's been on the market for seven years. Dr. Preuss had a professor at Vanderbilt University who made a similar recommendation, advising his medical students to never prescribe a drug that hadn't been on the market for at least five years.

Supplements have a far better track record. Yes, there have been rare problems with some of the supplements discussed in this book—problems that have been cited in the medical literature and that we present, so you can be aware of them. But overall, the supplements featured in *The Natural Fat-Loss Pharmacy* are far safer than prescription drugs. They meet the safety standards established for pharmaceuticals—and more.

They're natural. They are derived from food ingredients or herbs that have been in the food chain for hundreds or even thousands of years. You can't say that about new drugs.

They've been extensively tested for toxicity. Studies on laboratory animals have shown these supplements aren't toxic—they're unlikely to cause cellular damage or illness.

They've been used in research. They have been taken by people who participated in clinical trials, without significant side effects.

They've been on the market for a while. They have been taken for self-care by thousands and even millions of people, again without significant side effects.

As you'll see, there is an extensive discussion of the safety of each supplement that is recommended in this book—and, as you'll also see, each one is considered to be very safe. Of course, no substance is 100 percent safe—not even water. (Recent evidence shows, for example, that drinking too much water during long-distance running events like a marathon can create severe problems.) So we recommend that, for maximum safety, you take any weight-loss supplement only with the approval and supervision of your doctor. But rest assured: you can take the supplements recommended in this book with calmness and confidence, because it is very, very (did we say *very*?) unlikely they're going to harm you. The same can't be said about most drugs.

WHAT WE SAY TO THE NAYSAYERS

Of course, if you talk to your doctor (who is not likely to be well informed about using natural supplements for weight loss, fat loss, weight maintenance, *or* for better health), you might be told that even *if* these supplements are safe, they're not effective—and they're not going to help you lose weight. And your doctor might cite scientific research. Like this:

"The evidence for most dietary supplements as aids in reducing body weight is not convincing."

That's a statement by researchers who conducted a review of studies on weight-loss supplements, published in the *American Journal of Clinical Nutrition* (AJCN). Well, maybe those researchers didn't bother to read some of the other studies published in previous issues of AJCN—studies reported in this book (along with literally hundreds of others) that show many natural weight-loss supplements *do* work. For example:

- In two studies published in AJCN, green tea extract (EGCG) boosted calorie burning by 78 calories a day and improved weight and fat loss by 4 percent.

- In a long-term, two-year study reported in AJCN (and mentioned earlier in this introduction), CLA helped people lose 5 pounds of fat and gain 2 pounds of muscle.

- Another study in AJCN showed overweight women who got 5-HTP cut their calorie consumption by 1,341 calories a day.

And those studies are only the tip of a very large iceberg.

The problem with general conclusions about weight-loss supplements, like the negative statement we cited a moment ago, is that they're often made on the basis of a "meta-analysis" of lots of scientific studies—and are subsequently a mishmash of research and reasoning. And they often reflect a bias—an unstated but prevalent prejudice, learned at medical school—*for* prescription drugs and *against* natural supplements.

As you'll read in *The Natural Fat-Loss Pharmacy*, we examined all the research on each of the weight-loss supplements featured in the book—and came to a reasonable and practical conclusion about each one. In fact, we've included *only* those supplements that scientific research indicates can help you lose weight, lose fat, build muscle, and/or maintain weight. And that's why you won't find us talking about many of the overhyped weight-loss supplements on the market.

When you read the chapters in *The Natural Fat-Loss Pharmacy*, we think you'll see that—contrary to those researchers we quoted at the beginning of this section—the evidence for natural supplements as an aid to weight loss *is* convincing. If your doctor disagrees, ask him or her to read this book.

FAT LOSS AND WEIGHT LOSS:
WHY YOUR SCALE DOESN'T TELL THE WHOLE STORY

A core concept of this book is that *fat loss can be just as important as weight loss*—even if you're losing fat and not losing a lot of weight! To illustrate this point, we'll tell a tale of two dieters.

Before they start their weight-loss program, both dieters undergo DEXA, a sophisticated test that accurately measures body fat and what scientists call *lean mass*, most of which is muscle. After eight weeks, the scale shows that Dieter #1 has lost 6 pounds and Dieter #2 hasn't lost an ounce. Dieter #1 is the weight-loss winner, right? Not according to a second DEXA test.

Dieter #1, it turns out, lost 3 pounds of fat and 3 pounds of muscle.

Dieter #2, however, lost 3 pounds of fat—and gained 3 pounds of muscle. And Dieter #2—because she now has more calorie-burning muscle on her body—could continue to lose an *additional* 1 pound of fat per month. Not Dieter #1.

Which dieter would you rather be: hollowed out, calorie-compromised Dieter #1 or firmed up, calorie-clobbering Dieter #2? We think Dieter #2 has the edge. Unfortunately, most dieters are . . . Dieter #1.

Gilbert Kaats, PhD, executive director of the Health and Medical Research Center in San Antonio, Texas, and a colleague of Dr. Preuss, reviewed the results from several weight-loss studies in which 4,740 people were analyzed by DEXA.

He found that 21.9 percent of the dieters who had lost scale weight ended up with a *negative* change in body composition: that is, their overall ratio of muscle to fat got worse. They lost weight—but they lost more muscle than fat.

In contrast, 22.4 percent of dieters had no weight loss or even gained weight—but had an improved muscle-to-fat ratio.

As we asked a moment earlier: which dieters were better off? We think it's the folks with the improved muscle-to-fat ratio, not the people who lost "scale weight." And we think so for a couple of important reasons.

Breaking the cycle of yo-yo dieting. As we explained, when the typical dieter sheds pounds, he doesn't only lose *fat*. He loses fat *and* muscle. Muscle is metabolically active—pound for pound, it burns a lot more calories than fat. So the dieter loses muscle, burns fewer calories every day—and slowly but surely gains back the weight he lost . . . as fat! Weight regain is the fate of 95 percent of people who lose weight. Muscle loss during dieting is a major reason why.

Battling middle-aged spread. Starting in their thirties, most people begin to gain about 10 pounds per decade—the dreaded middle-aged spread. But at the same time they're gaining fat, they're also losing muscle—at the rate of about 5 pounds per decade. Reversing that trend is a way to beat the creep of pounds in middle age and later.

A trimmer, firmer body. People who lose fat and add muscle may not lose a lot of scale weight—but they do lose inches off their waists, hips, and thighs. They *look* a lot trimmer—and isn't that one of the main goals of weight loss?

More resistance to disease. Muscle is a major user of blood sugar, or glucose. People with a good muscle-to-fat ratio tend not to have high blood sugar levels—which can help prevent type 2 diabetes, high blood pressure, high cholesterol, arthritis, cancer, and even Alzheimer's disease.

What to Do

There are many ways to maintain muscle mass and reduce fat:

Exercise. Regular exercise is the most obvious, including weightlifting.

Limit refined carbs. Not overdoing it with refined carbohydrates (which are stored as fat) is another.

Stay away from trans fats. Also, stay away from trans fats found in baked goods like chips and cookies.

Take a natural supplement that improves muscle–fat ratio. An often

SUPPLEMENT SUPPORTER

PAMELA PEEKE, MD, MPH

www.drpeeke.com

Author, *Fight Fat After Forty* and *Body for Life for Women*; Pew Foundation Scholar in Nutrition and Metabolism and assistant professor of medicine, University of Maryland School of Medicine; adjunct senior scientist, National Institutes of Health; chief medical correspondent for nutrition and fitness, Discovery Health TV; medical commentator, CNN's *American Morning* and *Headline News*

In *Fight Fat After Forty*, Dr. Pamela Peeke told us about her breakthrough research at the National Institutes of Health, where she showed how chronic stress boosts levels of the hormone cortisol, blanketing our midriffs with more abdominal fat. (She's quick to point out that her research has *nothing* to do with the "quackery industry" of weight-loss supplements that claim to help you lose weight by reducing cortisol.)

In *Body for Life for Women*, Dr. Peeke presented proactive plans for the physical, emotional, and mental health of women of all ages—plans customized to the four "hormonal milestones" of a woman's life, from menarche to beyond menopause.

And in her medical practice, Dr. Peeke counsels women on how to lose fat,

overlooked but very effective way to maintain or improve muscle mass (particularly for people trying to lose weight): take one or more of the muscle-preserving, muscle-building supplements featured in this book, which include chromium, CLA, HMB, and BCAA.

HOW TO USE THIS BOOK

This isn't another diet book. It's a book you can use to improve the results you'll get following *any* diet.

This isn't another weight-loss plan. It's an approach you can use to im-

gain muscle, and increase their sense of self-worth. That advice might include taking a weight-loss supplement—*if* the woman already has in place a healthy blueprint for lifestyle change.

"Weight-loss supplements are an adjunct to weight control," she told us. "Healthy eating, appropriate physical activity, and stress management are the basics. Once they're in place, a supplement may have a role."

And, she points out, every person who is trying to lose weight should understand the possible downsides of taking a weight-loss supplement.

"It's just human nature to rely too heavily on a medication or supplement," she says. "People think they can forsake healthy lifestyle changes and just pop a pill—and that's not true."

Instead, says Dr. Peeke, people have to earn the right to take a supplement—by first proving that they're capable of putting lifestyle changes into place. Once those lifestyle changes *are* in place, a supplement may be appropriate.

"There is very provocative scientific research showing that certain weight-loss supplements could be an effective adjunct to losing weight," she says. And, she adds, some people may need those supplements more than ever.

"People are so much fatter now," says Dr. Peeke. "Long gone are the days when all most people had to do was drop 10 or 20 pounds to be healthier. Now, the American population is seriously overweight, with 40 percent of women and 30 percent of men obese. People need all the help they can get."

prove the results of *any* weight-loss plan—whether you're asked to follow it for a week, a month, or the rest of your life.

In fact, you'll find several of the authors of those plans—like bestselling diet authors Nicholas Perricone, MD (*The Perricone Weight-Loss Program*), Pamela Peeke, MD (*Fight Fat After Forty*, and *Body for Life for Women*), Mary Shomon (*The Thyroid Diet*), and Julia Ross (*The Diet Cure*)—featured in this book in "Supplement Supporter" boxes (see above) in which they explain their approach to weight loss *and* recommend one or more supplements they think could help out.

What's the best way to use this unique resource?

Read the book. You need inspiration and new ideas to aid weight loss. Give yourself the chance to find out about all the supplements featured in this book. We think you'll find them fascinating—and that once you know how potentially effective they are, you'll be ready to take action.

Consult Chapter 12. Once you've gotten the big picture, and have a feel for which supplements you think meet your needs, read Chapter 12, The Natural Fat-Loss Pharmacy Supplement Program. There you'll find a list accompanying each supplement, titled "Consider taking [supplement name] if . . ." Match those lists against your own goals.

You'll also find nine case histories from a top weight-loss doctor—case histories of people who've taken one or more supplements to lose weight. Read these stories, and see if you "see yourself" in any of them.

Make a decision. Next, make your decision about which supplement or supplements you want to take.

Talk to your doctor. And then talk to a doctor about what you're planning to do—and take supplements only with his or her approval and supervision.

Use the book as your one-stop weight-loss resource. You can use this book *with* any other weight-loss program. But you can also use it as *the* weight-loss program—because it includes comprehensive chapters on achieving a balanced diet and regular exercise. The diet chapter offers creative and easy ways to reduce calories—the core of any weight-loss program. The exercise chapter shows you how to use a pedometer (a device that measures steps) to get plenty of daily activity—the core of any program for not regaining the weight you've lost.

YOU CAN DO IT!

Many people suffer because of extra weight. If you're reading this, it's likely you're one of them. We want to help you—that's why we wrote this book.

Dr. Harry Preuss has been studying weight-loss supplements for decades. Bill Gottlieb has been writing about them for just as long. Together, we wrote *The Natural Fat-Loss Pharmacy* because we're firmly convinced that several nutritional supplements and herbs can be an effective addition to your efforts to lose weight. We think by reading this book you'll come to the same informed conclusion. There's no reason to deny yourself the help these supplements can offer. We wish you all success in your endeavors to achieve a trimmer, thinner body. We know you can do it. Particularly now that you've taken hold of that helping hand.

PART I

Fat Busters

Sip Your Fat Away

$\bullet$ EGCG (Green Tea Extract)

We humans drink more tea than any other liquid, except for plain old H_2O. And Bill Gottlieb does his part to keep tea number two.

Every morning before work, he makes himself a big pot of green tea (we'll talk in a minute about the differences among the three main types of tea—black, green, and oolong), and whether the variety he chooses is gunpowder, dragon well, or sencha, his daily ritual is always the same.

He fills a kettle with water and puts it on the stove to boil . . . spoons tea leaves into a mesh tea ball . . . places the tea ball in a ceramic teapot . . . fills the pot when the water boils . . . puts the pot on a tray . . . and carries the tray to his office, where he blissfully sips away while reading the morning paper.

And here are a few more tea-dious details about Gottlieb: he's fifty-three, five foot ten, and weighs 154 pounds—the same weight as when he graduated from high school.

Does drinking green tea every day for so many years have something to do with the fact that he's not suffering from middle-aged spread? A bunch of scientists in Taiwan might think so.

TEA DRINKERS ARE 20 PERCENT TRIMMER

This was the startling news published in the September 2003 issue of *Obesity Research* by Dr. Chih-Hsing Wu and a team of Taiwanese scientists at the National Cheng Kung University Hospital. They had studied more than one thousand men and women, with an average age of forty-eight, querying them about numerous "lifestyle characteristics."

Did they smoke? Drink alcohol? Coffee? What were their favorite foods and how often did they eat them? How much did they exercise? How much money did they make? And . . . how much tea did they drink a day, and for how many years had they been doing so?

But the researchers didn't only investigate habits. They also looked into hips. Specifically, they measured each person's percentage of body fat, and their waist-to-hip ratio, or WTHR. (WTHR is your waist measurement in inches, divided by your hip measurement. It not only shows the size of your belly, but also indicates how healthy you are: people who have a higher WTHR, storing more fat in their tummies, are at a greater risk for heart disease than people who store more fat in their hips and thighs.) The results from the Taiwanese study were remarkable.

Of those studied, 43 percent had been "habitual" tea drinkers for ten years or more, drinking about 15 ounces of tea a day.

The habitual tea drinkers had, on average, 19.6 percent less body fat than people who didn't drink tea regularly.

They also had slimmer waists, with a 2.1 percent lower WTHR.

No other lifestyle factor—whether or not they were smokers, snackers, sedentary, or high-salaried—correlated with a lower percentage of body fat. Tea was the likely ticket to leanness.

And only a few of those trimmer tea drinkers were regularly drinking Earl Grey, English Breakfast, or another variety of black tea. *Eighteen* of the habitual tea drinkers drank black tea. *Four hundred fifty-five* drank green or oolong. What's so special about those two varieties? To find out, let's take a quick trip to a tea plantation.

GREEN TEA:
LEAVING THE GOODNESS IN THE LEAVES

Black, green, and oolong tea all start the same way: as leaves on *Camellia sinensis*, an evergreen shrub that can grow to the height of a tree but is cultivated as a bush on tea plantations. A few times a year, the buds and the tender, young leaves at the top of the bush are picked and then dried on racks. But those dried tea leaves aren't ready for the teapot.

The next step is fermentation, as enzymes begin to break down other natural chemicals in the leaf. In black tea, fermentation is allowed to do its thing, producing a darkly colored, robustly flavored tea. But in green tea, fermentation is brought to a halt by heating: after drying, the leaves are lightly steamed or gently pan-fried in huge woks. Oolong tea is midway between black and green: a degree of fermentation is allowed to occur before the leaves are heated.

This seemingly slight difference in processing creates an enormous difference in the chemical composition—and the potential impact on your health—of green tea as compared to black. That's because the natural chemicals preserved in green tea leaves are a group of *polyphenols* containing *flavonoids* called *catechins*.

Let's define that trio of terms.

Polyphenols: Super-Protective Plant Chemicals

Polyphenols are polypopular—they get a lot of press. When you read about the health-giving power of the red in wine, the dark in chocolate, or the green in tea, you're reading about polyphenols. Plants produce polyphenols not because they want human beings to be healthier, but for their own protection: polyphenols are *antioxidants*, shielding plants from environmental harm.

A *flavonoid* is a type of polyphenol. There are five thousand of them, like the *quercitin* in kale, the *anthocyanins* in blueberries, and the *genistein* in soy.

Catechins (pronounced CAT-uh-kins) are a type of flavonoid found in high levels in green tea. (Green tea consists of 30 to 42 percent catechins, while black tea has 3 to 10 percent, with oolong in between.) Catechins aren't your everyday antioxidant: they're more powerful than antioxidant vitamins like A, C, and E in stopping the "free radical" damage to cells that can trigger chronic disease and speed aging. But that's not all catechins do.

In study after study in cell cultures, animals, and humans, they have been shown to help prevent, slow, or kill cancer cells—colon, breast, prostate, lung, skin, and others.

They can lower cholesterol, perhaps helping prevent heart disease. Ditto for high blood pressure.

They can lower blood sugar, perhaps helping prevent diabetes.

They can strengthen the immune system, helping to defuse viruses.

They can reduce inflammation, a harmful process linked to a host of diseases, from Alzheimer's to ulcers.

And—most important for this book—they can help burn calories and defuse fat making.

Scientists have isolated several catechins in green tea. But it's *epigallocatechin gallate*, or EGCG—the most abundant catechin in green tea—that we fat fighters are particularly interested in. An extract of green tea that contains high levels of EGCG may help you lose weight. And keep it off.

EXTRACT = EX-FAT

Let's move our green tea party from Taiwan to Switzerland. There, in 1999, Dr. Abdul Dulloo and his team of researchers at the University of Fribourg conducted an experiment on ten healthy men, publishing their results in the *American Journal of Clinical Nutrition*.

On three occasions, the men stayed for twenty-four hours in a "respiratory chamber"—an airtight room with all the comforts of a hotel (bed, armchair, table, TV, VCR, telephone, sink, and toilet). But this "hotel room" was inside a laboratory, where equipment measured differences between the air pumped into the respiratory chamber and the air pumped out, allowing researchers to calculate the exact amount of calories and fat the men burned while living in the chamber. During each of the three twenty-four-hour periods the men spent in the respiratory chamber, they took a particular set of pills with their breakfast, lunch, and dinner: (1) 50 milligrams (mg) of caffeine, (2) a combination of 90 mg of EGCG and 50 mg of caffeine, the amount of EGCG and caffeine in a cup of green tea, or (3) a placebo. The results?

The men burned a lot more calories when they took the EGCG/caffeine combo, compared to either the caffeine pill or the placebo—an average of 78 more calories over the twenty-four hours they spent in the chamber. The men also burned about 20 percent more fat on the EGCG/caffeine combo. How did the green tea extract incinerate extra calories and fat?

Dr. Dulloo theorizes that EGCG blocks the action of an enzyme that breaks down *noradrenaline* (NA), a hormone manufactured by the adrenal gland. NA functions as a neurotransmitter in the brain, stimulating the sympathetic nervous system, which controls heart rate, muscle tension, and the release of energy from fat. So when you take EGCG, the body's dominoes may fall like this:

EGCG keeps more NA in your brain . . . that extra NA triggers your metabolism to stay more active, thereby burning more calories . . . and the boost in NA also triggers extra fat burning.

Caffeine lends this process a helping hand, says Dr. Dulloo, blocking other enzymes that affect NA.

To add more evidence to their theory, Dr. Dulloo and his team measured the men's urinary levels of NA during each of the twenty-four hours they were in the respiratory chamber. And, sure enough, when the men took EGCG/caffeine supplements, their NA levels were higher than when they took either caffeine alone or the placebo.

Dr. Dulloo's conclusion: a green tea extract consisting of EGCG and caffeine has the potential to help people lose weight and fat. And he has another important opinion.

It's theorized that people who *eat* extra fat but don't *burn* extra fat (through increased exercise or some other means) develop a disordered appetite, craving and overeating fatty and other high-calorie foods. By burning fat, says Dr. Dulloo, a green tea extract may also help control the appetite of a person who typically eats a high-fat, high-calorie diet.

How Much EGCG Is Best?

The scientists in Switzerland aren't the only ones to have found that green tea extracts can burn extra calories and fat. A similar study was conducted by Dr. Sonia Berube-Parent and her team of researchers at Laval University in Canada and published in the *British Journal of Nutrition* in 2005.

The Canadian scientists wanted to answer two questions: Could they produce the same results as those from Switzerland—would an extract of EGCG/caffeine burn extra calories and fat? And if it did, what *dose* of EGCG/caffeine would work best?

To find out, the researchers studied fourteen healthy men, aged twenty to fifty, testing them on five separate days in a metabolic chamber (similar to a respiratory chamber). While in the chamber, the men took supplements three times a day that contained 200 mg of caffeine (from the herb guarana) and one of four different levels of EGCG: 90, 200, 300, or 400 mg. A few of the men took a placebo.

The answer to the first question was a qualified yes: the EGCG/caffeine extract increased calorie burning by an average of about 180 calories a day, compared to the placebo. But (unlike what happened in most of the other studies discussed in this chapter) it didn't boost fat burning. (Hey, one out of two ain't bad, especially when it's 180 calories a day—an amount of calories that could help you shed twenty-two extra pounds a year. Plus, many other studies *have* shown fat burning.)

The surprising answer to the question about dosage: 200, 300, and 400 mg doses did *not* burn any more calories than the 90 mg dose. Therefore,

EGCG: SAFER THAN ANTI-OBESITY DRUGS?

Dr. Sonia Berube-Parent and her Canadian colleagues at Laval University, as well as other researchers, theorize that EGCG works by stimulating the *sympathetic nervous system*, which controls heart rate, blood pressure, muscle tension, and fat burning. Dr. Berube-Parent points out that a green tea/caffeine combo might be *safer* than some of the anti-obesity drugs on the market, like Meridia (sibutramine), which also work in part by stimulating the sympathetic nervous system.

The problem with those drugs, she says, is not only can they increase calorie and fat burning—they can also boost heart rate and blood pressure. And in overweight folks, who are at a greater risk for developing heart problems, that boost, she says, "is a matter of concern for health professionals." (Not to mention the overweight folks themselves!)

"In this context," says Dr. Berube-Parent, the green tea/caffeine mixture (which studies show doesn't speed your pulse or raise your blood pressure) "seems to have potential as an effective alternative to these anti-obesity drugs."

Talk to your doctor about the possibility of using a green tea/caffeine extract as a natural alternative to prescription anti-obesity drugs.

says Dr. Berube-Parent, it's likely that 270 mg a day of EGCG is the "optimal concentration" to produce calorie burning.

She also points out that the EGCG/caffeine mixture didn't speed heart rate or significantly boost blood pressure levels—the cardiovascular symptoms experienced by some users of the now-banned ephedra, which also works by stimulating the sympathetic nervous system. (In fact, average blood pressure went up by only *one point*, from 122/74 to 123/75.)

Her final thoughts: An EGCG/caffeine mixture should be considered as a good addition to a weight-loss program, particularly one that includes nutritional smarts and regular exercise.

We couldn't agree more.

French Women Do Lose Weight

The studies in the respiratory and metabolic chambers were conducted over several twenty-four-hour periods. But what would happen if someone took a green tea extract for weeks or even months?

To find out, scientists in France studied sixty-three overweight women and seven overweight men for three months, giving them a green tea extract. Their results, published in the journal *Phytomedicine*, were very positive.

After three months on the extract, the group's average weight loss was 4.6 percent. And their waistlines shrunk by 4.5 percent.

Like the Canadian researchers, the French scientists note the people taking the supplement had no average increase in heart rate or blood pressure. A green tea extract, they conclude, might be a suitable natural supplement for people who are overweight, supporting their attempt to lose weight.

You won't hear us arguing with them.

Green Tea Extract and Exercise: Double Trouble for Fat

What happens when you take a green tea extract *and* you exercise? If you're a mouse that's been eating a high-fat diet, you lose a lot of weight. That was the finding of a team of Japanese scientists, reported in the journal *Medicine and Science in Sports and Exercise* in November 2005.

First, the researchers fed mice a high-fat diet. Next, they put the animals on one of three different regimens: exercise; green tea extract (GTE); or GTE and exercise.

The group of exercising mice lost 24 percent of that added weight.

The group of mice given GTE lost 47 percent of the weight they had gained.

But the group of mice that got GTE *and* exercised lost 89 percent of their extra pounds. (Okay, ounces.)

A similar study, reported in the October 25, 2005 issue of the *International Journal of Obesity*, produced the same results.

The researchers' conclusion: "The intake of tea catechins, together with regular exercise, helps to reduce diet-induced obesity."

It's great to know that a supplement you're taking to help you with weight loss may also boost the positive, pound-shedding effect of exercise.

Not Just Losing Weight but *Keeping* It Off

Another study shows that a green tea/caffeine extract may have an important role *after* you've lost weight—in helping keep the weight off. The experiment, conducted by Dr. Margriet S. Westerterp and her colleagues at Maastricht University in Holland, was published in the scientific journal *Obesity Research*. She studied seventy-six overweight men and women for four months. For the first month, they ate a very low-calorie diet, losing an average of 13 pounds. For the next three months, they ate a diet aimed at maintaining their weight loss. During that time, a group of the former dieters took an EGCG/caffeine supplement three times a day, before meals, for a total intake of 270 mg of EGCG and 150 mg of caffeine. Another group got a placebo. They were the unlucky group.

The group that took the green tea/caffeine extract *continued* to lose weight during the three months of weight maintenance, compared to the placebo group, which gained back an average of 40 percent of the weight they had lost.

But EGCG might not work to maintain weight loss . . . if you drink a lot of coffee. Oddly enough, people who took the EGCG/caffeine supplement but also got *more* than 300 mg a day of caffeine from their diet *didn't* maintain their weight loss as effectively as people who took EGCG/caffeine and had a dietary intake of caffeine *under* 300 mg. So if you drink two or more cups of coffee a day, an EGCG/caffeine supplement might not help you keep your weight off. (The researchers don't know why.)

But for those who don't have too much caffeine in their diet, a green tea extract might be a good choice, says Dr. Westerterp. "I recommend an EGCG/caffeine supplement to support weight maintenance after weight loss," she told us. "Of course," she added, "one must also eat healthy food at an intake matched to one's daily requirement for calories."

EGCG: SLAYER OF FAT CELLS

Researchers call them *adipocytes,* and you call them . . . well, what you call them might not be printable here.

We're talking about *fat cells.*

Robbins. He recommended green tea for weight loss, just like Oprah. I went out and bought some—a powdered variety that I mixed with hot water. I drank about 32 ounces of that green tea for a month. I didn't lose a pound, but the tea seemed to give me the mental clarity to stick with my weight-loss program—to begin eating the way I needed to eat to lose weight."

Using a customized meal replacement program, and under the strict supervision of her doctor, Mary Jane quickly lost weight: 152 pounds in less than a year. "But I believe the spark could have been green tea," she says. "They say it's an amazing mental tonic. And it certainly seemed to give me the clarity to stay focused on losing weight. A clarity I'd never had before."

After losing her weight, Mary Jane maintained her weight *and* lost an additional 20 pounds—simply by making healthier food choices and changing her lifestyle. She continued to use meal replacements. With foods she loved and wanted to eat, like cupcakes and pizza, she followed a "two-bite" rule, so she could enjoy but not overdo. She sought out and added new and delicious fruits to her diet. She exercised regularly. (Today, she's an aerobics teacher.) And, in many other innovative ways, she learned how to think, feel, and live as a thin person—or, as she told us, a *passionate* person, challenged and fulfilled by life. In fact, she plans to write a book about her experience, so she can help others achieve their weight-loss goals. Mary Jane offers her perspective and advice about weight loss at www.maryjanemedlock.com.

Once upon a thinner time (twenty years ago, when 74 percent fewer Americans were overweight), scientists thought people were born with a set number of fat cells, which stayed constant throughout life. Fat cells might grow larger but you couldn't grow more of them.

Now, however, it's understood that two things can happen when you get fatter: fat cells can get bigger *and* you can develop new ones. Conversely, when you lose weight, fat cells can shrink *and* you can get rid of them— which means that anything that can kill fat cells might help you lose weight. EGCG does just that.

In an experiment conducted by Dr. Clifton Baile and other researchers at the University of Georgia, fat cells exposed for twenty-four hours to EGCG died at a much higher rate than fat cells exposed to a "control" chemical. And the longer the exposure to EGCG, the more fat cells died. After three or four days of exposure, more than 50 percent of the cells were dead. (In fact, so many cells died that the researchers couldn't get an accurate count.)

Dr. Baile also found that EGCG stopped *adipogenesis*—the creation of new fat cells. Again, the higher the levels of EGCG the newly forming cells were exposed to, the less likely they were to reach maturity. "EGCG may prove to be a valuable natural product in the treatment of obesity," writes Dr. Baile, in the June 2005 issue of *Obesity Research*.

OOLONG, TOO

Scientists have also looked at the fat-beating power of oolong tea, which contains less EGCG than green but more than black.

A study on oolong tea was conducted by Dr. William Rumpler, at the USDA Human Nutrition Research Center in the U.S. and his colleagues at the Department of Nutrition at the University of Tokushima in Japan, and published in the *Journal of Nutrition*.

Twelve men, twenty-five to sixty years old, were given one of three different beverages on three separate days: full-strength oolong tea; half-strength oolong tea; and water with 270 mg of caffeine. On each of those days, the men (like those in the Swiss and Canadian studies) lived in a laboratory, where the researchers measured the amount of calories and fat they burned.

And, sure enough, the men drinking the full-strength tea burned 67 percent more calories a day than when they were drinking just water. They also burned 12 percent more fat.

Oolong tea consumption, concludes Dr. Rumpler, could help people maintain lower levels of body fat.

Fighting Fat

A study on oolong tea *and* a green tea extract was conducted by Dr. Ichiro Tokimitsu and his colleagues at the Health Care Products Research Laboratories of the Kao Corporation, and published in the *American Journal of Clinical Nutrition* in 2005.

For their twelve-week study, the researchers divided thirty-five men into two groups, giving one group a daily bottle of oolong tea enriched with 690 mg of green tea catechins, while a second group got oolong tea containing only an extra 22 mg of green tea catechins. At the beginning and the end of the study, the researchers weighed all the men and also measured a number of indicators of body fat. It was a lot leaner being green.

Compared to the 22 mg group, the 690 mg group lost 1.5 percent more weight; had a 1.5 percent greater decrease in BMI (body mass index, a measure of fatness); lost 2 percent more from their waists; had a 3.7 percent greater drop in body fat mass; had a 7.9 percent greater decrease in total fat area . . . and had a 7.5 percent greater reduction in subcutaneous fat (fat right underneath the skin).

Important: This was a three-month study, which means it took a little bit of time for the fat-reducing effects of EGCG to become obvious. "It takes time for body fat reduction to become apparent with EGCG," Dr. Tokimitsu told us. "Therefore, it is important to *continue* to ingest tea catechins, and not expect instant results."

Less LDL

There was another measurement of body fat the researchers found intriguing: lower levels of the blood fat LDL, or low-density lipoprotein.

LDL is the "bad" cholesterol that forms the clumps of arterial plaque that narrow arteries, increasing your risk of a heart attack or stroke. Specifically, the researchers measured MDA-LDL, a particularly nasty type of LDL that is a common component of arterial plaque.

The men getting the higher levels of tea catechins had lower levels of MDA-LDL.

These results, says Dr. Tokimitsu, suggest that catechins can help lower not only a person's level of body fat, but also their risk for heart disease and "various lifestyle-related diseases."

Let's take a look at some of those "lifestyle-related diseases" like heart disease, cancer, and diabetes (and some other diseases that are just plain bad luck) and see how EGCG might help.

EGCG TO THE RESCUE?

We don't want to tout EGCG as some kind of snake oil, able to cure whatever ails you. It can't do that. *No* pill—natural supplement or prescription drug—can do that. However, scientists have conducted hundreds of experiments investigating EGCG, and many of them demonstrate its proven or potential power to prevent and treat disease. Here's an A-to-Z recap of some recent research highlighting the health-giving goodness of EGCG.

Aging. Maybe the biggest fear about aging is the fear of literally losing your mind—the gradual fading of memory, clarity, and concentration, the looming possibility of developing Alzheimer's or suffering a stroke. Good news for our aging population: researchers in Israel have found that EGCG can prevent the death of neurons, or brain cells. And in a study published in the *Journal of Neurochemistry* in June 2005, they found EGCG can actually help "rescue" neurons *after* they've been damaged. Their findings, they say, "suggest that EGCG may have a positive impact on aging and neurogenerative diseases to retard or perhaps even reverse the accelerated rate of neuronal degeneration."

Allergies. In laboratory tests on human cells, EGCG blocked the production of histamine and immunoglobulin E (Ige), two compounds that trigger allergic responses. The study was conducted by researchers in Japan and reported in the *Journal of Agricultural and Food Chemistry.*

Alzheimer's disease. Researchers at the University of Southern Florida gave EGCG to mice genetically programmed to develop Alzheimer's-like brain changes. The extract prevented much of the brain injury associated with

NATURAL FAT-LOSS PHARMACY SUCCESS STORY

Four Women Who Lost 25 Pounds Each

Elizabeth Jones is a certified clinical nutritionist in Vermont. When she counsels overweight clients, she works with them to break food addictions, lower stress, eat more fruits and vegetables and low-fat protein foods, exercise, chew thoroughly, drink more water, take antioxidant and fish oil supplements—and use green tea extract.

"EGCG is not a stand-alone therapy for weight control, but it is a very valuable adjunct, helping control appetite and burn fat," she told us. "I give it to all of my overweight clients. One client said she'd rather drink the tea—but that's an awful lot of tea, and she gave up and started using the supplement."

In the last year, Jones has advised four women to take EGCG, and each of them lost at least 25 pounds.

"These clients were women aged forty-seven, sixty-five, fifty, and fifty-five," she says. "The sixty-five-year-old had gone through an enormous amount of stress. Her husband had a heart bypass operation and she was a caretaker for her dying parents. She started to eat a lot of comfort foods and stopped exercising. Over five years, she gained 50 pounds. But once she was eating right and exercising and taking her supplements—including green tea extract—the pounds just dropped off and she returned to her normal weight."

Jones says that even if EGCG didn't help with weight loss she would probably advise her clients to take it. "It's anticancer, lowers cholesterol, and is a powerful antioxidant," she told us. "It's just a wonderful substance."

Alzheimer's disease, including a 54 percent decrease in the formation of the beta-amyloid plaques that are the primary indication of Alzheimer's. "These data," wrote the researchers in the *Journal of Neuroscience* in 2005, "raise the possibility that EGCG dietary supplementation may provide effective prophylaxis [prevention] for Alzheimer's disease."

Bladder cancer. In laboratory research from scientists at UCLA, EGCG induced "cell adhesion" in bladder cancer cells, making them less mobile and therefore less likely to grow and spread. The researchers are currently conducting a clinical study with EGCG on patients with bladder cancer to see if it can help prevent a recurrence of the disease.

Breast cancer. When scientists at Boston University School of Medicine combined EGCG with breast cancer cells, the substance changed the "gene expression profile" of the cells, making them much less virulent. Their research was reported in the December 2005 issue of the *Journal of Nutrition*.

In other research in 2005, scientists at the University of Alabama at Birmingham found that EGCG could stop the development of "estrogen receptor negative" breast cancer cells—a type of breast cancer that spreads fast and is hard to treat. In their positive assessment of the power of EGCG, the researchers assert: "EGCG possesses anticarcinogenic effects against ER-negative breast cancer cells" and could be developed as "a novel and pharmacologically safe chemopreventive agent for breast cancer prevention."

Cervical cancer. Researchers studied eighty-eight women with chronic cervical inflammation (cervicitis) or cervical dysplasia (a precancerous condition), giving some of them EGCG and some other treatments. Of the women receiving the extract, 69 percent improved—human papillomavirus (HPV), which is linked to cervical cancer, was reduced or eliminated; the size of cervical lesions decreased; and the abnormal cells of dysplasia vanished. Of the women not receiving EGCG, 10 percent improved. The research was reported in the *European Journal of Cancer Prevention* in 2003.

Cholesterol problems. Researchers divided 220 adults with high cholesterol into two groups. For twelve weeks, one group received a green tea extract enriched with theaflavins, a potent polyphenol formed during the fermentation of black tea. The other received a placebo. In the extract group, total cholesterol decreased by 11 percent and "bad" LDL cholesterol by 16 percent. There was little change in the placebo group. The research was conducted by scientists at the Vanderbilt University Medical Center in Tennessee (Dr. Preuss's training grounds) and reported in the *Archives of Internal Medicine* in 2003.

Colon cancer. Researchers at Columbia University in New York found that EGCG inhibits a number of key processes involved in the proliferation, or spread, of human colon cancer cells. "EGCG may be useful in the chemo-prevention or treatment of colorectal cancer," they wrote in the September 2005 issue of *Biochemical and Biophysical Research Communications.*

Diabetes. In type 2 diabetes, blood sugar isn't effectively absorbed by the cells and circulates in the bloodstream, creating metabolic havoc. The most common complications of type 2 are a nightmare: heart disease; stroke; nerve damage leading to foot or leg amputation; blindness; and kidney dis-ease. In research in India, scientists found that EGCG protected the red blood cells of diabetics from the types of changes that can cause complica-tions. "We hypothesize" that catechins like EGCG "may provide some pro-tection against the development of long-term complications of diabetes," they write in a 2005 issue of *Clinical and Experimental Pharmacology and Physiology.*

Flu. In cell cultures, EGCG stopped three different types of influenza virus from replicating. The research was conducted in South Korea and reported in the November 2005 issue of *Antiviral Research.*

Fungal infections. Researchers in Japan tested EGCG against the common fungal infection *Candida albicans*—and it cut fungal growth by 91 percent. And when the researchers used EGCG *with* standard antifungal drugs, it improved the performance of the drugs. Combined treatment with catechin "allows the use of lower doses of antimycotics [antifungal medication]," they write in the February 2004 issue of the *Journal of Antimicrobiotic Chemotherapy.* "It is hoped," they continue, "that this may help avoid the side effects of antimycotics."

Heart attack. In laboratory studies, researchers in the UK found that EGCG can reduce the number of heart cells that die after a heart attack and also speed up the postattack recovery of heart cells. The research was published in the FASEB (Federation of American Societies for Experimental Biology) journal in 2005. Other research shows that EGCG can inhibit *platelet aggregation*—the clumping of blood cells that can lead to the formation of blood clots that cause heart attacks and strokes.

More evidence on green tea and heart disease: Researchers in Japan analyzed the green tea intake of 109 people with heart disease and 94 people without the problem. Those without heart disease drank an average of 5.3 cups of green tea a day; those with heart disease, 3.5 cups. "The more green tea patients consume, the less likely they are to have cardiovascular disease," conclude the researchers, in the July 2004 issue of the *Japanese Circulation Journal.*

Helicobacter pylori. This stomach-based bacterial infection can cause ulcers. Scientists in Japan took strains of *H. pylori* that had been resistant to certain antibiotics and put them in cell cultures with EGCG and previously unused antibiotics. EGCG *and* the new antibiotics were more powerful in killing *H. pylori* than the new antibiotics alone. "These results indicated that EGCG may be a valuable therapeutic agent against H. pylori infection," the scientists wrote in 2003 in the journal *Current Microbiology*.

Immune weakness. Researchers in the Department of Medical Microbiology and Immunology at the University of South Florida College of Medicine exposed *macrophages* (infection-fighting white blood cells) to a particularly nasty substance: cigarette smoke condensate. The macrophages became a lot weaker, unable to produce certain infection-fighting chemicals like interleukin-6, and unable to stop a pneumonia virus. But when the macrophages were treated with EGCG, they were able to produce those infection-fighting chemicals *and* resist the virus. The study was reported in 2002 in the journal *Clinical and Diagnostic Laboratory Immunology*.

Leukemia. Scientists at the Mayo Clinic took cancer cells from patients with chronic lymphocytic leukemia (CLL) and put them in a test tube with EGCG—and a lot of the cancer cells died. When some leukemia patients at the clinic found out about these results, they started taking over-the-counter EGCG supplements, without telling their doctors. But a few of those patients couldn't keep their self-care therapy under wraps for long—because their worsening leukemia started to get better! The doctors reported these cases in the December 2005 issue of *Leukemia Research*. As this book was being written, the Mayo Clinic had started a clinical trial to test EGCG on patients with early-stage CLL.

Lou Gehrig's disease (amyotrophic lateral sclerosis). This neuromuscular disease progressively weakens and destroys motor neurons, the cells that connect the brain and skeletal muscles. Korean researchers gave EGCG to mice genetically altered to develop ALS. Compared to similar mice not getting EGCG, the EGCG mice got symptoms later in life and also lived longer. "EGCG could be a potential therapeutic candidate for ALS as a disease-modifying agent," the researchers wrote in the December 12, 2005 issue of *Neuroscience Letters*.

Lung cancer. When Chinese researchers combined lung cancer cells with EGCG, the extract decreased the power of the cells to invade noncancerous areas. Their study was reported in the April 2005 issue of *Biomedicine and Pharmacotherapy*.

Possible anticancer mechanism: Researchers from the UK and Spain showed that EGCG binds to and inhibits the enzyme DHFR, which plays a role in the growth of both normal and cancer cells and is an established target for the anticancer drug methotrexate. They reported their study in *Cancer Research* in 2005.

Metabolic syndrome. This disorder—also called syndrome X and insulin resistance—afflicts one in four Americans. It's a deadly combination of overweight, high blood pressure, high triglycerides (a blood fat), low levels of HDL ("good" cholesterol), and insulin resistance (a prediabetic condition of abnormal blood sugar metabolism, with higher than normal blood levels of insulin and blood sugar). When laboratory animals bred to have excess weight and insulin resistance were fed EGCG, the animals lost weight and had lower blood levels of blood sugar and insulin. The study was conducted by researchers in Japan and reported at a meeting of the American Physiological Society.

Pancreatic cancer. Researchers at Case Western Reserve University in Ohio found that EGCG fights pancreatic cancer by damaging the *mitochondria*, or energy-generating cores, of cancer cells, and thereby causing *apoptosis*, or "programmed cell death." Their research was reported in the May 2005 issue of *Carcinogenesis*.

Prostate cancer. Italian researchers studied sixty-two men, aged forty-five to seventy-five, with high-grade prostatic intraepithelial neoplasia (PIN), a premalignant condition that leads to prostate cancer in about 30 percent of cases. For one year, thirty-two of the men received a green tea extract, while thirty received a placebo. At the end of the year, only one man in the green tea group was diagnosed with prostate cancer. Nine in the placebo group—the predicted 30 percent—got the disease. The doctor who led the study says that his data suggests that nine out of ten cases of prostate cancer in high-risk men, such as African-Americans and those with a family history of the disease, might be prevented by EGCG. The research was presented at the annual meeting of the American Association for Cancer Research in 2005.

Skin cancer. In a laboratory study, dermatologists in the UK found that EGCG could prevent UVA-caused damage in skin cells—the same kind of sun damage that may contribute to the development of skin cancer. As part of the same study, the scientists asked ten people to drink green tea, subjecting samples of their cultured cells to twelve minutes of UVA radiation before and after the tea drinking. There was much less DNA damage to the cells *after* the tea was consumed. This research was reported in the February 2005 issue of *Photodermatology, Photoimmunology and Photomedicine*.

Stomach cancer. Researchers in Japan combined EGCG with four "cell lines" of stomach cancer cells. In each case, EGCG stopped the cells from multiplying. The more EGCG, the stronger the effect. The study was published in the April 2005 issue of the *Biological and Pharmaceutical Bulletin*.

Stroke. Japanese researchers induced strokes in two groups of experimental animals, one given EGCG and one not. EGCG reduced the extent, intensity, and negative effects of the stroke. The researchers' conclusion: "Daily intake of green tea catechins efficiently protects the penumbra [the area of the brain affected by the stroke] from irreversible damage due to cerebral ischemia [stroke] and consequent neurological deficits." This research was reported in the June 2004 issue of *Medical Science Monitor*.

HOW TO USE EGCG

Okay: enough about problems *other* than overweight. Let's talk about the best way to use EGCG to lose weight and fat, and keep it off.

Take EGCG right before meals. In most of the studies on EGCG/caffeine and weight loss, the participants took the supplement three times a day, before meals. That makes sense, because EGCG/caffeine supplements work, in part, by telling your body to burn more calories and fat—and you might as well start with the calories and fat you just ate!

(However, if you take EGCG for other therapeutic effects—such as cancer prevention—your best bet might be taking it first thing in the morning, before you eat. That was the finding of researchers at the Arizona Cancer Center at the University of Arizona in Tucson, who studied EGCG absorption in thirty healthy people. They found that the EGCG in green tea extracts was absorbed 3.5 times better when taken first thing in the morning, before eating, than when taken with breakfast.)

Take the right amount. Based on her research on weight maintenance with EGCG, Dr. Westerterp recommends a supplement that provides a daily intake of 575 mg of tea catechins, with 325 from EGCG, and 100 mg of caffeine.

Don't rely on tea. Why not just drink three or four cups of green tea a day to get that amount of EGCG and caffeine? Well, there's nothing wrong with drinking green or oolong tea regularly—just ask Gottlieb. It's relatively inexpensive, tasty, and probably really good for you. But most of the studies on weight loss and weight maintenance were conducted with green tea *extracts*. So that's the proven and reliable way to get plenty of EGCG into your system—and to get the calorie-burning, fat-busting results you want. Plus, in a study comparing the antioxidant power of green tea extracts versus green tea—extracts won.

Researchers at UCLA gave thirty people either a green tea extract, green tea, or black tea, with each source standardized to deliver the same amount of EGCG. Eight hours later, they tested the blood of the tea drinkers for antioxidant activity. Compared to the people drinking green or black tea, those getting the green tea extract had a "significant increase in plasma antioxidant activity," said the researchers in the December 2004 issue of the *American Journal of Clinical Nutrition*.

Pick a product with the right amount of EGCG and caffeine. Look for a product that meets Dr. Westerterp's recommendations for EGCG and caffeine. There are many on the market. A few possible choices among widely distributed brands include:

Teavigo 300 with Guarana, from GNC. This product includes a highly purified green tea extract (Teavigo) that has been successfully used in experiments on laboratory animals to prevent weight gain and reduce body fat, and also has been extensively tested for safety. Two pills a day provide 270 mg of EGCG and 180 mg of caffeine.

Schiff Green Tea Diet. Each pill provides 225 mg of green tea extract, 90 mg of EGCG, and 50 mg of caffeine, amounts that are quite close to Dr. Westerterp's recommendations.

Thermo Green Tea Caps by Universal Nutrition, which provide 90 mg of EGCG and 50 mg of caffeine per pill.

IS EGCG SAFE?

Human beings have been drinking green tea for thousands of years. If there were any side effects, we'd probably know by now.

But human beings *haven't* been taking EGCG—a highly purified extract of green tea—for thousands of years. That's a recent development. Is EGCG safe?

According to two studies published in the journal *Food and Chemical Toxicology*, in December 2005—the answer is yes.

Researchers tested EGCG (Teavigo), feeding extremely high levels to laboratory animals and then examining their cells for genetic damage. There was

ENVIGA: THE REAL THING?

Can Coke help you lose weight? Okay, not Coke exactly—but a new product from Coca-Cola: Enviga, a 5-calorie beverage that contains EGCG and caffeine.

In a scientific study conducted at the University of Lausanne in Switzerland, researchers gave three 12-ounce cans of Enviga a day to thirty-two normal-weight adults. The thirty-two people drank Enviga between meals for three days—and burned 60 to 100 calories more per day than when they weren't drinking the beverage.

Should you consider Enviga a smart way to get your daily dose of EGCG and caffeine? Well, if you like the flavors (green tea, berry, and peach) enough to think that you'll reliably drink three cans a day, day after day (at a cost of about $4.00 a day), why not? Three cans of the drink deliver 270 milligrams of EGCG and 300 milligrams of caffeine—similar to the amount that studies show is optimal for burning calories and maintaining weight loss.

none. In another study, conducted by the same researchers, laboratory animals were fed large doses of EGCG for thirteen weeks, with no adverse effects.

What about us humans?

For four weeks, researchers at the University of Arizona gave up to 800 mg a day of EGCG (in single or divided doses) to thirty-two healthy people. A similar group received placebos. There were no more "adverse events" like headaches or nausea in the EGCG group than there were in the placebo group, and there was no significant change in blood chemistry in the EGCG group.

"We conclude," write the researchers, in the August 2003 issue of *Clinical Cancer Research*, "that it is safe for healthy individuals to take green tea polyphenols in amounts equivalent to the EGCG content in 8–16 cups of green tea once a day or in divided doses twice a day for 4 weeks."

Another study on people was conducted in Switzerland and reported in the July 2004 issue of the *International Journal of Vitamin and Nutrition Research*. EGCG (Teavigo) was given daily for ten days to thirty-six healthy men—either 200, 400, or 800 mg. The researchers write that every level of EGCG was "safe and very well tolerated."

Add to these safety studies the fact that EGCG has been on the market for quite a while without any hue or cry over side effects, and it appears to be a very safe supplement.

Pregnancy Precautions

As with *all* natural supplements, however, EGCG shouldn't be taken by pregnant or lactating women (except with the approval and supervision of a gynecologist). In fact, the scientists who discovered one possible mechanism for the anticancer powers of EGCG—binding to and inhibiting the action of the enzyme DHFR—say that same mechanism might also reduce folate absorption. And a lack of folate has been linked to birth defects.

This caution is completely speculative: there is no proven link between EGCG and birth defects. But even a speculative link is reason enough for pregnant women not to use the extract.

Is the Caffeine Okay?

Most doctors don't forbid their patients with heart problems to drink coffee or tea. But, to be extra safe, if you've experienced heart difficulties of any kind, you should talk to your doctor before taking an EGCG/caffeine combination.

A Product Not to Take

Although it's not available in America (and even hard to find on the Internet), stay away from Exolise, a green tea extract from a French company that was sold as an over-the-counter weight-loss drug. Writing in the French journal *Gastroentérologie Clinique et Biologique*, a team of researchers reported that thirteen people who took Exolise developed elevated liver enzymes (a sign of liver problems). In twelve people, the enzymes returned to normal when they stopped taking the extract, but one person went on to develop liver toxicity, a much more serious problem.

Does this result indicate that *all* over-the-counter EGCG products are potentially harmful? No, says Dr. Preuss, who thinks the preponderance of evidence points to the safety of products containing EGCG.

Lose Body Fat—Without Dieting or Exercise

- CLA (Conjugated Linoleic Acid)

Picture, if you will, a ruminant—an animal that chews its cud, a wad of food regurgitated from the rumen. (This is going to get a lot more appetizing very soon, so hang in there.)

Picture a cow. Or a sheep. Or a goat. The ruminant is probably grazing (ever see a cow do much of anything else?)—munching on grass, hay, or some other extreme-fiber food that is *really* hard to digest. Ruminants, however, don't have access to Alka-Seltzer. So to make life and lunch a little bit easier, Mother Nature provided ruminants with a four-part stomach.

Part one—the mega-gallon rumen—is populated by billions of microbes, which help out with digestion. In the process, those busy little bacteria break down two fatty acids (building blocks of fat) called *linoleic acid* and *linolenic acid* into a unique fatty acid found almost nowhere else in nature but in ruminants: *conjugated linoleic acid*, or CLA.

Scientists discovered CLA in 1978. And it's been impressing them ever since.

In studies on cells, laboratory animals, and people, CLA has shown it has the potential to:

- Stop cancer from spreading.

- Strengthen the immune system.

- Improve asthma.

- Calm inflammation.

- Balance blood sugar.

- Lower high cholesterol and high blood pressure.

And—like a dieter's dream come true—studies also show that CLA can melt body fat and build muscle without *calorie cutting or exercise.*

Sound too good to be true? You won't think so after you read the rest of this chapter.

THE DISCOVERY OF CLA

Rewind to 1979, the year when an accident at the Three Mile Island nuclear power plant almost deep-fried Pennsylvania, Iranians took Americans hostage, and Russians invaded Afghanistan. Some good things happened, too.

One of them was in a laboratory at the Food Research Institute of the University of Wisconsin at Madison. There, a team of researchers, led by Michael Pariza, PhD, were diligently investigating . . . grilled beef patties. That's right—guys in white lab coats were dissecting hamburger meat. They wanted to confirm (or perhaps disprove) a recent finding that was troubling food scientists—and food eaters—across America and around the world: that grilling beef could produce *mutagens*, chemicals that can warp the molecules of a cell's genetic material, possibly leading to cancer.

Unfortunately for those who think charcoal briquettes are a food group, the Wisconsin scientists found mutagens in grilled hamburger. But they also found something they didn't expect: a chemical that *reduced* the formation of mutagens.

They found CLA.

And, they theorized, CLA might help block cancer. They were right. Only it turned out that CLA can do a lot more than tame tumors.

CLA vs. Cancer, Cholesterol—And Body Fat

Thousands of scientific studies have highlighted the health-giving potential of CLA. Many of the breakthrough studies—research exploring previously uncharted areas of CLA's impact on health and disease—were conducted in Dr. Pariza's laboratory.

In 1987, he and his colleagues used CLA to stop the development of skin cancer in laboratory animals.

In 1994, they showed that CLA could reduce the inflammation generated by an immune system in overdrive.

That same year, they found that CLA-fed rabbits on a high-fat diet had much lower levels of "bad" LDL cholesterol than rabbits not fed CLA.

And, in 1997, they showed that mice fed a diet supplemented with CLA ended up with 60 percent less body fat and 14 percent more lean body mass (LBM, which is mostly muscle) than mice not fed CLA. In that same study, cellular analysis showed CLA might stop fat from being deposited in fat cells, help break down fat cells (lypolysis), and help burn up fatty acids in both fat cells and muscle cells.

Well, with that finding, obesity researchers around the world went ape . . . or, more accurately, they went mice, hamster, rat, chicken, and pig. In research conducted in Japan, America, Canada, Australia, and Poland (to name drop a few nations), curious scientists conducted experiments on the body fat of various species of laboratory animals, feeding some a CLA-enriched diet, while others didn't get CLA. In most of those studies, the CLA animals ended up with much less body fat and much more lean body mass than animals not fed CLA.

BAD FOR FAT

It was time for scientists to see if CLA could perform the same fat-busting, muscle-building magic in us humans. CLAbracadabra—it did!

Fat loss—in the overweight. Researchers in Norway studied forty-seven overweight people for twelve weeks, dividing them into five groups. (As you'll see, the Norwegians aren't only good at cross-country skiing, raising reindeer, and frolicking on fjords. They're also number one when it comes to proving that CLA is bad for fat.) One group got a placebo. The other four groups got various levels of CLA per day: 1.7, 3.4, 5.1, or 6.8 grams (g). The researchers measured body fat mass (BFM) at the beginning and at the end of the study.

Over the twelve weeks, the placebo group didn't lose any BFM. (In fact, they added some.) But most of those getting CLA lost a lot of fat. For instance, those getting 3.4 g of CLA lost almost 4 pounds of body fat. And all four CLA groups had a small increase in lean body mass.

"The beneficial effects of CLA with regard to body fat mass and lean body mass . . . are promising," wrote the researchers in the *Journal of Nutrition* in 2000.

Over the next five years, that promise was fulfilled. Bigtime.

Fat loss—in the "spare tire" of middle-aged men. Swedish researchers studied twenty-four men, aged thirty-nine to sixty-four, all of whom were— well, let's put it semi-politely, like the researchers did—"abdominally obese." Fourteen of the men got 4.2 g of CLA for four weeks, while another ten got a placebo.

The CLA guys lost an average of half an inch off their waistlines. The placebo guys also had a tad of fat whittled off their waists—eight hundredths of an inch, to be exact.

"CLA supplementation," wrote the researchers, in the *International Journal of Obesity* in 2001, "may decrease abdominal fat."

Gutsy conclusion.

Fat loss—in young, healthy exercisers. In 2001, researchers in Norway studied twenty healthy, young people of normal weight who exercised four or more hours every week. The researchers divided them into two groups, giving one group 1.8 g of CLA daily and the other a placebo for twelve weeks. After twelve weeks, the body fat of the CLA group decreased from 21.5 percent of their weight to 17 percent. The placebo group? No change at all. These results, the researchers wrote in the *Journal of International Medical Research* in 2001, "support a body fat reducing effect of CLA."

Fat loss—after weight loss. Researchers at Maastricht University, in Holland, studied fifty-four people who had been on an extremely low-calorie diet for three weeks, losing an average of 15 pounds. For the next thirteen weeks, the dieters took either CLA or a placebo. Over those weeks, both the CLA and the placebo groups regained weight—from 22 to 48 percent of the pounds they'd shed. But the placebo group gained back 42 percent more fat, as compared to the CLA group, who gained most of their weight back as "fat free mass," or muscle.

Gaining weight back after three weeks on a super-rigorous crash diet is bad enough. Gaining it back as fat is adding insult to injury. But gaining weight back as firm muscle rather than flab . . . well, that's a regain a lot of us could live with.

It's Not Unanimous

But not all the CLA studies on fat loss and muscle gain were positive. Some researchers found CLA didn't subtract fat or add muscle. Why not?

Was the dose of CLA too low? Were the scientists using the wrong type of CLA? Were too few people being studied to show a "significant" (as scientists say) statistical result? (It's hard for researchers to detect numerically meaningful changes when they study small groups of people.) Were the studies too brief—not enough weeks or months to show a measurable result? And what about the safety of CLA? Would people participating in a longer study suffer side effects from the supplement not seen in shorter studies?

Those were some of the questions posed by Dr. Jean-Michael Gaullier, a scientist at Scandinavian Clinical Research, near Oslo, and his team of researchers from various medical centers in Norway and from the Norwegian Food Research Institute. To answer them, Dr. Gaullier and his colleagues conducted two one-year studies on CLA—one right after the other, using the same group of more than one hundred people. Two years of research on a hundred-plus people usually produces results that scientists consider *conclusive*—it's not likely those results will be contradicted by future studies.

And Dr. Gaullier's results couldn't be better news for people who *don't* want to diet but *do* want trimmer, leaner bodies.

ONE YEAR, ONE CONCLUSION: CLA DEFEATS FAT

A total of 180 men and women participated in Dr. Gaullier's first one-year study. They were healthy—they didn't have diabetes, heart disease, cancer, or any other serious health problem. They were teens, seniors, and in-betweeners—from eighteen to sixty-five years old. Genderwise, XX outnumbered XY, with 149 women and 31 men.

But all the participants had one thing in common: they were overweight.

Body mass index (BMI, a measure of overweight) ranged from 25 to 30. (What does that "index" mean in everyday terms? A person five feet, seven inches tall and weighing 160 pounds—slightly overweight—has a BMI of 25. At 192 pounds, that same person has a BMI of 30.)

At the beginning of the study, the participants were randomly divided into three groups. One group received a daily dose of six soft gel capsules of CLA in the form of *free fatty acids*. A second group received the same dose of CLA in the form of *triacylglycerol*. (These are technical terms for two different types of CLA that are commonly found in supplements. Dr. Gaullier wanted to see if one type was more effective than the other.) A third group received a placebo—fake, look-alike pills that contained olive oil rather than CLA.

And here's the most interesting feature of the study: the participants weren't asked to make any changes in their lives except to take two CLA supplements with each meal.

No cutting calories.

No additional exercise.

Just take the pills.

Measuring Success

To figure out whether or not CLA was working to cut fat and add muscle—and whether or not it was safe—the researchers took a few different measurements at the beginning and the end of the study, and every three months or so.

Body composition. Were there changes in the percentages of body fat mass (BFM) and lean body mass (LBM)? Because this was the "primary outcome" researchers wanted to measure, they used sophisticated and highly accurate technology: dual-energy X-ray absorptiometry (DEXA), which pinpoints fat tissue, lean tissue, and bone, and is the "gold standard" in determining body composition.

Weight. Were the participants losing weight or not?

BMI. Was their BMI increasing or decreasing?

Adverse effects (AEs). What kinds of side effects were they having, if any?

Blood samples. Was blood chemistry—twenty-six different factors, from hormones to minerals to blood sugar to cholesterol—changing for good or ill?

Compliance. Were the participants actually taking the supplements? (If you don't take the pill—for whatever reason—it isn't going to work.)

One hundred fifty-seven people stuck with the study for a year, with some dropping out for various reasons (like getting pregnant).

And the winners were . . . the people taking CLA.

8 Percent Less Fat, 2 Percent More Muscle

More fat loss. At the end of the twelve months, the CLA group had an average decrease in body fat of 8 percent more than the placebo group.

More muscle gain. Likewise, they had an increase in lean body mass 2 percent greater than that of the placebo group.

On average, the CLA group lost 4½ pounds of fat and gained 1½ pounds of muscle. The placebo group saw little or no change in either fat or muscle.

More weight loss. People taking CLA didn't just lose fat and gain muscle—they also lost weight: an average of 3 pounds. The placebo group didn't lose any.

Better BMI. The BMI of the CLA group decreased slightly. The BMI of the placebo group didn't budge.

No diet or exercise required. And those results didn't depend on diet and exercise. No matter what people ate and how much they exercised—CLA worked.

Fast results. It didn't take a whole year for CLA to trigger those effort-free changes. In fact, most of the fat loss and muscle gain occurred in the first six months of taking CLA. "Our studies showed that, in some cases, maximum fat loss occurred after three months of supplementation," Dr. Gaullier told us. "In other cases, it took six months."

Overweight women do best. There were two subgroups that benefited the most from CLA: those with the highest BMI, and women. That's probably because, pound for pound, women have a higher percentage of body fat than men, says Dr. Gaullier. And fat is what CLA gets rid of.

There was little difference between the CLA mixtures: both free fatty acids and triacylglycerol worked equally well.

TWO YEARS, TWO CONCLUSIONS: CLA WORKS—AND IT'S SAFE

Dr. Gaullier continued his study because he wanted to evaluate the safety of CLA over a really long time. After all, he points out, CLA is already on the market, so it's crucial to know whether or not it's safe to take for years on end.

Of the 157 study participants, 134 continued to take CLA for another twelve months. Dr. Gaullier's conclusion about CLA's safety after twenty-four months was the same as his conclusion after twelve: CLA is safe. Very safe.

Almost No Side Effects

As with the first twelve months of the study, there were almost no side effects from taking CLA. Seven people suffered from mild digestive problems now and then, like stomachache, loose stools, or nausea.

Is CLA Bad for Your Heart?

People who took CLA had slightly increased levels of lipoprotein-A, or Lp(a), a fat-protein particle similar to LDL (low-density lipoprotein)—and, like LDL, linked to heart disease. Is CLA a mixed blessing, reducing body fat while hurting your heart? Dr. Gaullier doesn't think so.

Yes, he says, the effect of CLA on heart health isn't completely understood and will require more study. But, he points out, changes in other blood fats more directly linked to heart disease—total cholesterol, LDL, and heart-helping HDL—were "very small" and "within the normal range,"

CLA: NOT JUST ONE THING

In this chapter, we talk about CLA as if it's *one thing*, a single substance. But it's really a *group* of similar things.

Think of CLA as . . . well, as a baseball team—the CLA Dodgers.

All the CLA Dodgers are on the same team, wear the same uniform, and play the same game—but they're still individuals. Just so, the CLA team is a group of individual *isomers*—chemicals composed of the same elements, in the same proportions, but each with a slightly different arrangement of atoms.

And just as a baseball team has a pitcher, a centerfielder, and a shortstop, each with a different skill set, so the various isomers of CLA do different tasks. One isomer specializes in fighting body fat. Another battles cancer cells. And sometimes CLA isomers execute a double play, working together to accomplish a result.

The two most biologically active isomers are those most commonly used in CLA supplements. They're named using a scientific shorthand that describes their molecular structure: *cis*-9, trans-11 and *trans*-10, cis-12. (We'll spare you the chemistry lesson: *yawn*-1, zzz-2.)

Luckily, there are no free agents in nature. You can keep those CLA isomers on *your* team for the rest of your life.

---

indicating *no* increase in risk for heart disease among those who took CLA.

A few months after Dr. Gaullier's study was published, Swedish researchers, writing in the November 2005 issue of the *British Journal of Nutrition*, reported that CLA supplements increased C-reactive protein, another possible "marker" for increased risk of heart disease.

"This is not a problematic finding," says Del Dorscheid, MD, an assistant professor of medicine at the University of British Columbia, in Vancouver, and an expert in CLA. "The increase was within the normal range, and was not clinically or medically relevant."

Like Dr. Gaullier, Dr. Dorscheid thinks CLA is quite safe.

"CLA has been studied on over six thousand people and there have been no significant adverse effects reported—no acute allergic reaction, no acute physiological distress," he says. "And that lack of side effects was again demonstrated in Dr. Gaullier's study, which tracked usage for two years."

An Increased Risk for Diabetes?

Researchers at Uppsala University in Sweden found that overweight men given 3.4 g of CLA a day showed a 19 percent increase in *insulin resistance*— the hobbling of the hormone insulin as it tries to move blood sugar out of the bloodstream into cells, and an early warning sign of type 2 diabetes. Should you be concerned? No, says Dr. Gaullier.

During his two-year study, no one taking CLA developed diabetes. And other studies have shown that CLA supplementation can *decrease* blood sugar in diabetics, possibly helping to control the disease.

He also points out that the men in the Swedish study who developed insulin resistance were taking a CLA "isomer" that wasn't used in his study. Those receiving the combination of two CLA isomers used in his study did *not* develop insulin resistance.

Long-term supplementation with CLA, he concludes, does not cause diabetes.

SAY NO TO THE YO-YO

Perhaps the most important finding of Dr. Gaullier's two-year study, however, is that the people on CLA *didn't gain back their fat, and they didn't lose any additional muscle.*

And that's crucial for anyone who is trying to *maintain* weight loss. Dr. Gaullier explains:

When the typical dieter (or person using a weight-loss drug) sheds pounds, she doesn't just lose *fat*. She loses fat *and* lean body mass, or muscle. Muscle is metabolically active—pound for pound, it burns a lot more calories than fat. So the dieter loses muscle . . . burns fewer calories every day . . . and slowly but surely gains back the weight she lost.

That's the sad scenario suffered by nine out of ten dieters. That's nine people—multiplied by a couple of million—who might want to take CLA.

"CLA may be beneficial in preventing weight regain, which is part of the yo-yo effect often observed with many diet plans," says Dr. Gaullier. That was certainly what happened to those who took CLA in his study.

"CLA supplementation prevented loss of lean body mass during weight reduction," says Dr. Gaullier, thereby "reducing the risk of weight increase."

The bottom line (not to mention your waistline) on CLA? You can use it to:

- Tone your body—without diet and exercise.

- Combine CLA with diet and exercise for even more effective weight loss.

- Stop weight regain after a diet.

How can one natural supplement do all that?

How CLA Deflates Fat

Nobody knows for sure exactly how CLA frustrates fat cells. But there are several likely explanations, says Dr. Pariza. CLA probably stops dietary fat from getting into fat cells by blocking the action of lipase, an enzyme that helps with the job. CLA may also affect the development of new fat cells. And it may help burn up fatty acids in muscle.

HOW TO USE CLA FOR FAT LOSS

Taking CLA is very straightforward.

Amount. The people in Dr. Gaullier's study used 3.4 g a day—and you should too, if you want the same results. But pay close attention to the label

GOOD-MOOD MEDICINE
FOR THE DIET BLUES

You're dieting so you can lose weight and feel better about yourself—but right now you feel *terrible*.

You've got hunger pangs and headaches. Sometimes you're restless and irritable, and sometimes you're lethargic and depressed. You can't concentrate. And you definitely don't want to think about . . . sticking . . . to this lousy diet . . . one more lousy day . . .

Don't stop dieting. Start taking CLA.

That was the recommendation from two studies on dieters reported in 2003 at a symposium on CLA and health in Kansas City. Researchers found that overweight dieters who took CLA had a significant reduction in the diet blues, compared to dieters getting a placebo. CLA, they concluded, makes it easier to stay on a diet.

"When people try to lose weight there are all kinds of physiological changes that can produce lethargy, depression, and other psychological symptoms," says Del Dorscheid, MD, an assistant professor of medicine at the University of British Columbia in Vancouver, and an expert on CLA. "Taking CLA can alleviate all that, giving dieters an increased sense of wellness, and helping them stay on their diets."

on the supplement. For example, a pill may be 1 g (1,000 mg) but contain only 80 percent CLA, thereby delivering 800 mg of CLA. Four of those pills per day would equal an intake of 3.2 g. You may have to do a little math to make sure you're getting enough.

Timing. The people in Dr. Gaullier's study took two pills, three times a day, with meals. Other CLA experts say that taking pills twice a day is fine. What's most important is that you actually *take* the supplements, on a schedule that works for you. Many people find they're more likely to take supplements *every* day if they take them *fewer* times per day—once or twice, rather than three times.

Side effects. What if you're one of the very few people who have digestive problems when they take CLA? "Reduce the amount of CLA you're taking by half," says Dr. Gaullier. "If the side effects persist, stop completely for a few days and then start again, at full dosage. If, at that point, the problems don't disappear, you're not someone who can take CLA."

Products. As with all the supplements discussed in this book, Dr. Preuss recommends you use the same brand or brands of CLA that were used in the studies that proved its effectiveness.

In his study, Dr. Gaullier used Tonalin CLA, which is a fifty–fifty mixture of two CLA isomers.

Tonalin CLA is found in many brands of CLA, including products from these companies:

Blue Bonnett	Natural Factors
Bodyonics	Nature's Bounty
Challenge	Nature's Way
Country Life	Next Step Nutrition
Doctor's Trust	Now
Dymatize	Optimum Nutrition
EAS	Prolab
FoodScience of Vermont	Pro Performance
GNC	Puritan's Pride
Good 'n' Natural	Safeway Select
HDT	Source Naturals
Human Development Tech	Swanson
Iron-Tek	Vitabase
Jarrow Formulas	Vitamin Shoppe
Life Extension	Vitamin World
Life Service Supplement	Wellness Partners
Natrol	Your Life

Food won't do it. Do you *have* to take a supplement—couldn't you just eat more foods rich in CLA? Nope. The best sources of CLA are meat

NATURAL FAT-LOSS PHARMACY SUCCESS STORY

Fat Loss After Pregnancy

It was 1994, and Cindy Dorscheid, twenty-eight years old, had just had her first baby. Like most new mothers, she'd gained some extra fat during her pregnancy—fat she didn't want to keep around. How to get rid of it? She didn't have time to exercise. She didn't want to go on a diet—especially since she was nursing. And that's when she read about CLA, a supplement that scientific studies showed might banish extra fat—a *natural* supplement that would be safe to take while she nursed her baby.

"So she took CLA," says Del Dorscheid, MD, an expert in CLA—and Cindy's husband. "Her waistline got smaller. The tops of her arms lost their extra fat. She didn't lose any weight—CLA typically doesn't do that. But she lost size in areas that made her feel better about herself—because she looked better and her clothes fit better."

But, says Dr. Dorscheid, his wife's more positive outlook after taking CLA might not only be a reflection of her trimmer body—CLA *itself* may improve mood.

"My wife found that if she ran out of CLA—because we had toddlers and couldn't get to the store, or for whatever reason—she wouldn't feel as good emotionally. And not only would her mood worsen, but her asthma and allergies would come back."

Dr. Dorscheid is a respiratologist—a specialist in asthma and breathing disorders—so he was particularly intrigued by the link between his wife's respiratory symptoms and CLA. Recently, he conducted a breakthrough study showing that CLA can normalize asthma in people with mild to moderate disease. (Please see page 64 for more information about the study.)

"My wife has continued to take CLA for the last twelve years," he told us, "because she knows that when she's taking it her shape is more firm and less fat.

"I've lived with her for all the years that she's been taking it, and I have certainly seen what it can do—and that's motivated me to research CLA and actually prove whether or not it has medical benefits. It does."

and milk from ruminant animals. And the average intake from those sources is 212 mg a day for men and 151 mg for women. You need to get about *twenty times* that amount of CLA to lose fat and weight. You can only do that with a supplement. "You would probably rather take a few pills than eat several pounds of cheese every day," says Dr. Gaullier.

BEYOND FAT LOSS

For more about CLA than you want to know, take a quick trip to www.wisc. edu/fri/clarefs.htm. There, Dr. Pariza and his colleagues maintain a database of references to every new scientific study about CLA—and there are a lot of them.

In 2005, for example, nearly three hundred studies were published on CLA, including studies in which CLA slowed the spread of cancer cells, helped stop bone loss in postmenopausal women, calmed the inflammation of asthma, was linked to lower rates of colon cancer, and boosted immune function. Let's look at some of that research.

Strengthening immunity. Scientists at the Rowett Research Institute in Aberdeen, Scotland, gave 3 grams of CLA a day to twenty-eight healthy men and women and then measured their immune function. They had an increase in blood levels of two antibodies that fight bacteria, viruses, and other invaders. "This is the first study to show that CLA can beneficially affect immune function in healthy human[s]," the researchers wrote in the *European Journal of Clinical Nutrition* in April 2005.

Normalizing asthma. Mild to moderate asthmatics who took 4 grams of CLA a day for twelve weeks had a *complete* normalization of their airways, as measured by their response to methacholine, a drug that constricts airways and is used to determine whether or not a person has asthma.

SUPPLEMENT SUPPORTER

NICHOLAS PERRICONE, MD

Author, *The Perricone Weight-Loss Program*, *The Perricone Promise*, *The Perricone Prescription*, and many other anti-aging and beauty books; adjunct professor of medicine, Michigan State University School of Medicine

The dermatologist and bestselling author Nick Perricone, MD, is pro-youth and anti-wrinkle. But he's also anti-inflammation. *Very* anti-inflammation.

Inflammation, he explains, is the protective response of the immune system to infection and irritation. Sunburn is an example of *acute* inflammation. But inflammation also comes in a *chronic* variety, visible only under a microscope. And chronic inflammation is a likely cause of many chronic diseases, like heart disease, diabetes, cancer, and Alzheimer's. The insult to those injuries: chronic inflammation can also make you fat.

"Body fat is never present without inflammation," Dr. Perricone told us. In fact, he says, chronic inflammation is the *very basis* of not only body fat, but also of out-of-control appetite, food cravings, food addiction, and the inability to lose excess weight. To counter chronic inflammation, Dr. Perricone recommends his three-part, anti-inflammatory weight-loss program.

You maximize your intake of ten anti-inflammatory foods, like wild salmon, fruits, and avocados. You incorporate elements of an anti-inflammatory lifestyle, like regular exercise and stress reduction. And you take a variety of anti-inflammatory nutritional supplements. Including CLA.

"CLA is a powerful aid in the prevention and treatment of obesity," says Dr. Perricone. He points out that the nutrient can block the absorption of fat into fat cells, reduce the size of fat cells, and prevent muscle loss. "What could be more exciting or encouraging than a supplement that shrinks body fat while increasing and preserving lean muscle mass?" he asks. He recommends 1,000 to 4,000 milligrams of CLA a day, in one or two doses, taken with meals.

"This is a profound finding," says Del Dorscheid, MD, who conducted the study at the University of British Columbia in Vancouver. "Mild to moderate asthmatics have very poor compliance with the inhaled steroids that are used to treat the disease—only about a third take their medication regularly, because of fears of side effects." So, he says, finding a safe, natural product that can effectively treat mild to moderate asthma is potentially of "tremendous benefit."

Treating overweight . . . and osteoporosis. Believe it or not, scientists are finding that overweight and osteoporosis (bone loss) may have the same cause: fat cells (adipocytes) replacing bone-forming cells (osteoblasts)!

By slaying fat cells—something done very handily by CLA—you might be helping to prevent osteoporosis. "Natural products" such as CLA may be "effective treatments for osteoporosis," say researchers at the University of Georgia in Athens.

More evidence: In a study published in the June 2005 issue of the *Journal of the American College of Nutrition*, researchers at the University of Connecticut found that the higher the intake of CLA (from both food and supplements), the higher the bone mineral density in postmenopausal women.

Fighting cancer. In a study reported in the journal *Anticancer Research* in November/December 2005, researchers in France reduced the growth of various types of human cancer cells—breast, lung, colon, prostate, and skin—by exposing them to CLA.

In other recent studies on CLA and cancer, high dietary intake of CLA from lean meat was linked to a lower risk for colon cancer; and CLA blocked a growth factor that fuels breast cancer cells, leading scientists at Ohio State University to conclude "CLA might serve as a chemo-therapeutic agent in human breast cancers."

Heart disease. Irish researchers fed mice a diet to produce clogged arteries (atherosclerosis) and then fed them a diet supplemented with either CLA or saturated fat.

"CLA supplementation did not simply prevent progression" of atherosclerosis, they wrote in the September 2005 issue of *Atherosclerosis*, "but in-duced almost complete resolution."

They found that CLA turns off genes that cause inflammation—one cause of the development of artery-clogging plaque—and also kills cells in arterial plaque.

3

Stop Your Body from Manufacturing Extra Fat

- HCA (Hydroxycitric Acid)

If you're an aficionado of Indian cuisine—curries, chutneys, chapattis, and the like—you're no doubt familiar with *tamarind*, a delightfully sour spice derived from the dried rind of the tamarind fruit. A variety known as the *malabar tamarind* (*Garcinia cambogia*, to you botanists out there) is particularly popular in the western coastal areas of southern India and in Sri Lanka, an island off India's southeast tip. The malabar tamarind is typically used to add a sour, fruity flavor to pork and fish curries. But it has talents beyond the tasty.

Locals have long noted (for a couple of millennia) that foods spiced with the malabar tamarind not only taste great but also are more filling—they *really* satisfy appetite. And extracts of the spice have been used in traditional medicine, to treat indigestion and heart disease.

In the late 1960s, plant scientists began to wonder about and investigate the rind of this unusual fruit. Chemical analysis revealed it to be a rich source of a fruit acid somewhat similar to the citric acid found in oranges and lemons. (*Acid* is a technical term in chemistry, where substances are categorized as either acid, alkaline, or neutral.) But this acid turned out to be a rare and unique biochemical, found mainly in *Garcinia cambogia* and two of its botanical cousins.

Its name: *hydroxycitric acid*, or HCA.

Its unique powers: turning down your appetite, and turning your body's fat-making machinery to *Slow*.

WHAT IS HCA?

To help you understand how HCA works to aid weight loss, we're going to be your tour guides on one of those fantastic voyages—you know, where you shrink to microscopic size and visit the inside of the body. In this case, you're going to get *extremely* small—about one-tenth the diameter of a strand of hair, or the size of a cell. Step this way.

Interfering with Fat

The body has about 10,000,000,000,000 cells. (That's 10 *trillion*, the kind of number you only see in scientific treatises and budget forecasts.) There are about two hundred different types of cells and each is a "specialist" in a particular area of the body: the heart, liver, muscles, bones, or other organs and tissues. But no matter where cells reside, they have a couple of features in common.

They're covered by a cell membrane. They contain cytoplasm, a watery fluid. At the center is a nucleus, home to DNA and RNA. And doing the heavy lifting are thousands of *enzymes*, a type of protein.

Enzymes are catalysts: they break apart and put together molecules, speeding up chemical reactions inside the cell. In this chapter, the enzyme we're particularly interested in is *citrate lyase*.

Citrate lyase plays a key role in a process that fuels the cell, called the Krebs cycle (named after the German biochemist Hans). In the Krebs cycle, simple sugars (carbohydrates) are broken down into molecules that can be put back together as fatty acids (fat). And in our fantastic voyage, here's what's really fantastic about HCA:

HCA blocks a portion of citrate lyase from breaking down citric acid into acetyl coenzyme A, thereby decreasing the formation of cholesterol and triglycerides, the building blocks of fatty acids. In other words, HCA lowers the level of a key enzyme that helps sugars and starches turn into fat!

That's not a hopeful theory. That's a scientific fact, with plenty of research to back it up, including several studies conducted by Dr. Preuss and his colleagues. We'd like to tell you in detail about two of those studies, because the results show just how uniquely effective HCA can be in helping you lose weight.

WELCOME TO INDIA (OR IS THAT THINDIA?)

The two studies were conducted in Andhra Pradesh, a state in southeast India. They were overseen by Dr. Preuss and several of his colleagues: a professor in the Department of Pharmacy Sciences at Creighton University Medical Center, in Nebraska; a professor in the Department of Statistics at the University of Connecticut; and two professors from India, one from the Department of General Medicine at ASR Academy of Medical Sciences, and one from the Department of Pharmacy at Andhra University.

In the first study, Dr. Preuss and his co-researchers looked at thirty people, ranging in age from twenty-one to fifty. They were healthy but overweight, with a BMI between 30 and 50. (For example, a five-foot-four-inch woman weighing 170 pounds has a BMI of 30; a woman of the same height weighing 290 pounds has a BMI of about 50. A healthy BMI is below 25.)

All the participants engaged in a sensible, moderate weight-loss program, eating a diet of 2,000 calories a day and walking thirty minutes, five days a week. The study lasted eight weeks. Dr. Preuss and the other scientists examined the participants at the beginning of the study, after four weeks, and at the end of the study. Each time, they measured several parameters. Among them were:

- Body weight

- BMI

- Two blood fats: cholesterol ("bad" LDL and "good" HDL) and triglycerides

- Appetite reduction

- Leptin (a hormone generated by fat that helps regulate appetite and metabolism: lower levels are better for weight loss)

- Serotonin (a brain chemical, or neurotransmitter, that influences appetite: higher levels are better for weight loss)

- The urinary levels of several breakdown products of fat (higher urinary levels of these "metabolites" indicate that more fat in the body is being burned up, or oxidized)

The study participants were divided into two basic groups. The first group received HCA—a special form called HCA-SX, or Super CitriMax, in which the HCA is hooked up to the minerals potassium and calcium for better absorption. (At the end of this chapter, where we discuss how to maximize the effectiveness of HCA, we'll explain why all HCA supplements are definitely *not* created equal.) The second group received a placebo, a look-alike pill. Neither group knew if they were getting HCA or the placebo. But after two months, the difference was obvious—inside the body and out.

HCA Wins Hands Down—And Pounds Down

The people taking HCA outscored the placebo group in all of the factors measured.

Weight loss. Over the eight weeks of the study, the placebo group lost an average of 3 pounds. But the group taking HCA lost 12 pounds—*four times* as much weight.

BMI. The average BMI in the placebo group fell by 1.7 percent. In the HCA group, it fell by 6.3 percent.

Blood fats. Those taking HCA had a 20 percent boost in HDL, the "good" cholesterol that carries fats away from the bloodstream to the liver. The placebo group had an 11 percent increase.

The HCA group had a 12 percent decrease in LDL, the "bad" cholesterol that deposits fat in arteries. The placebo group had no change.

The HCA group had an 18 percent drop in triglycerides. The placebo group, 9 percent.

Appetite. Over the eight weeks, the placebo group had a slightly *higher* intake of food, eating an average of 2.8 percent more food at each meal. Meanwhile, the HCA group gained greater control over their collective appetite, choosing to eat an average of 4 percent *less* food during each meal.

Leptin. The placebo group had a tiny drop in leptin levels of 0.3 percent. (Remember, lower levels are a plus for weight loss.) In contrast, those who took HCA had a drop of 37 percent.

Serotonin. The placebo group did have a significant boost in serotonin levels, at 21 percent. But they were outpaced by the HCA group, at 40 percent. It's a well-known fact that stress—anxiety, worry, tension—can cause overeating. Higher serotonin levels are calming, perhaps leading to better appetite control.

Fat burning. Those taking HCA had an average 200 percent increase in urinary levels of fat metabolites—a sure indication their bodies were burning more fat. The placebo group had almost no increase. The HCA group probably burned more fat because their bodies were making less—so they started using stored fat for fuel.

The results of this study were so positive that Dr. Preuss and his colleagues decided to conduct another, larger study.

HCA VS. FAT: ROUND 2

The number of people was doubled, with sixty healthy, overweight people participating. Everything else about the two studies was pretty much the same, with one group getting HCA and the other getting a placebo. The results were published in the journal *Diabetes, Obesity and Metabolism* in 2004. And—for people who want an effective weight-loss supplement to assist them in a sensible program of diet and exercise—the results were extremely encouraging.

Beyond the Plateau

The HCA group lost an average of 10 pounds. The placebo group, 3½.

And the HCA group didn't just lose *more* weight than the placebo group. They *continued* to lose weight throughout the eight weeks of the study, in contrast to the placebo group. In other words, the HCA group never found themselves on the dreaded "weight loss plateau"—that metabolic stall where you're cutting calories and exercising regularly, but your body refuses to shed any more pounds.

The HCA group had a decrease in BMI of 5 percent. The placebo group, 2 percent.

As for fat burning: the HCA group had a 100 percent increase in "fat metabolites" in their urine, while the placebo group had a 21 percent increase.

The HCA group had a drop in leptin of 40 percent. The placebo group, 2 percent.

A Petite Appetite

Perhaps the most remarkable result was in appetite control. The placebo group had *no* change. But the HCA group had a 16 percent reduction in the amount of food they ate per meal! Why the big drop?

It may be biochemistry. HCA stops carbs from forming fat. Those carbs are then stored in the liver and muscles, a process that may send satiety signals to the brain, saying, "We don't need any more *fuel*, so tell [insert your name] not to eat any more *food*!"

Or it may be brain chemistry. Increased levels of serotonin may put a brake on the impulse to overeat.

Whatever the cause—body, brain, or both—it's a fact that HCA helps control appetite: it helps you feel full rather than hungry or deprived, so you don't overeat. That's great news for dieters. And there's more good news— for dieters' hearts.

Blood fats were lowered in the HCA group, with 13 percent lower LDL, and an 8 percent boost in HDL. The placebo group had no significant changes.

The conclusion by Dr. Preuss and his colleagues, as stated in the study: HCA is an "efficacious weight-management supplement." Translated into everyday language: HCA works! And Dr. Preuss isn't the only scientist who thinks so.

A HISTORY OF EFFECTIVENESS

There are many other scientific studies—conducted at universities and research centers in America and around the world—that show HCA can effectively aid weight loss.

HCA can help you stay on your diet. In 1995, Spanish scientists published a study on HCA in the journal *Investigación Médica Internacional*. For the study, they put thirty-five overweight people (twenty-six women and nine men, with an average age of thirty-seven) in two groups, giving one group HCA and the other a placebo. Both groups went on a calorie-restricted diet for the eight weeks of the study: 1,000, 1,200, or 1,500 calories a day, depending on their degree of overweight.

The first important finding: most of those taking the HCA found they

NATURAL FAT-LOSS PHARMACY SUCCESS STORY

Postmenopausal Weight Loss

Linda R., fifty-three, works for an accounting firm in southern California. She went through menopause at forty-nine and, she says, the pounds started creeping on. At five foot six and weighing 170 pounds, she started to feel like she *had* to lose weight.

"But now that I've gotten a little bit older, I realize that it's harder to lose weight," she told us. "Clearly, my metabolism has changed. In my fantasy, I would love to go back to my twenties or thirties, when it was so easy to lose extra weight. But reality says no."

To lose weight, she decided to cut out all the "bad carbs" she'd read about, like sugar, pastries, and white bread, and gradually introduce more high-fiber good carbs, like whole-wheat bread and pasta. "I didn't want to go on any extreme diets," she says. "I just wanted to try to eat healthier." She also started walking a few times a week. Then her brother-in-law told her about HCA. And she started taking it.

"HCA definitely affected my appetite," she says. "It was subtle—not so dramatic that I noticed it instantly. But it's been definite—slow and steady and healthy and easy. I'm ecstatic that I don't have the cravings that I used to, and that it's easier to practice proper portion control. I even go out to restaurants and it's so great not feeling that I have to eat *everything* on my plate. When I'm full, I stop. That's delightful."

After starting HCA, Linda lost 20 pounds in four months. What does she think about her new, slimmer body?

"I feel like I'm looking good," she says. "People will say to me, 'How'd you do it, Linda? How did you lose that 20 pounds? You look great.' And I say, 'I've been eating healthy and exercising—and taking HCA.' "

could stick with their diet, while most of those taking the placebo weren't able to eat the smaller amounts of food.

And after eight weeks, those taking HCA had lost an average of 9 pounds, while those taking the placebo had lost only 3 pounds. In other words, HCA triggered *three times* the amount of weight loss!

The HCA group also had significant decreases in total cholesterol (18 percent) and triglycerides (26 percent), compared to small changes in the placebo group. And they had a significant drop in blood pressure, going from an average of 127/82 to 117/74.

The scientists conclude: HCA is "effective as a coadjuvant [a treatment that lends a helping hand to the main therapy] in weight loss in obese subjects, since it enables them to decrease the intake of high-calorie foods."

Eat less—without feeling hungrier. In 2002, Dutch researchers at the University of Maastricht published results of a study on HCA in the *International Journal of Obesity and Related Metabolic Disorders.* They studied twenty-four people: twelve men and twelve women, with an average age of thirty-seven, and an average BMI of 27.5 (the equivalent of a five-foot-ten-inch person weighing 192 pounds). All the participants got HCA for the first two weeks of the study, then a placebo for the next two weeks, then HCA for the last 2 weeks. During the periods when they took HCA, the study participants ate anywhere from 15 to 30 percent less food—without feeling hungry or deprived.

Get rid of that gut—even if you don't lose weight. In a study from Japan, published in 2001, researchers put forty overweight people on a diet for eight weeks, with half receiving HCA and the other half a placebo. In this study, the people who got the HCA didn't lose more weight than the placebo group. But they did lose significantly more *fat*—including extra "visceral" or abdominal fat. That type of fat is both unattractive *and* unhealthy: it's been linked to an increased risk of heart disease and diabetes.

OTHER HEALTH BENEFITS

Because HCA blocks the creation of fat from carbohydrates . . . and reduces appetite . . . and lowers cholesterol and triglycerides . . . and boosts serotonin, taking the supplement may help with conditions other than over-weight.

Lowering the risk of heart disease in diabetics. Diabetes isn't the biggest killer of diabetics—that dishonor goes to heart disease. Diabetics tend to have heart attacks earlier in life than nondiabetics and those attacks are more often fatal. If people with diabetes can reduce their levels of artery-clogging cholesterol, they can reduce their risk of heart disease and their risk of death. HCA may help them do just that.

In a study from India, published in the *Karnataka Journal of Medical Sciences* in 2001, researchers gave HCA for two months to fifty-two people with type 2 (adult-onset) diabetes. At the end of the two months, those with the highest total cholesterol—200 to 280 mg/DL—had an average 11 percent reduction. Those with slightly lower but still high levels of total cholesterol—140 to 200 mg/DL—had an average drop of 9 percent. The participants also saw a significant increase in "good" HDL and a significant decrease of "bad" LDL cholesterol. As an added benefit, HCA helped control the diabetes itself, lowering blood sugar levels by an average of 11 percent. The researchers conclude that HCA shows "a significant favorable effect" on cholesterol in type 2 diabetics.

Lowered risk of diabetes, too. Dutch researchers gave rats either HCA or no HCA before two laboratory procedures that mimicked eating and digesting a meal (infusing sugar into the stomach or small intestine).

The rats getting HCA had a much slower rise in blood sugar. And a much slower fall—blood sugar remained circulating for two hours in the HCA rats, compared to twenty minutes in the non-HCA rats.

This reduction in the peaks and valleys of blood sugar levels is *exactly* what nutritional experts counsel people to achieve by eating more fiber, or low glycemic foods, or fewer refined carbohydrates, or more protein—strategies designed to keep blood sugar and insulin levels on an even keel and help prevent type 2 diabetes.

"If we can reduce the peaks and valleys of postmeal blood sugar and insulin with HCA, then HCA might have some application in diabetes, slowing progression to type 2 diabetes and helping to prevent obesity in diabetics," said Peter W. Wielinga, one of the researchers who conducted the study, in an interview with the American Physiological Society.

The study was reported in the June 2005 issue of the *American Journal of Physiology-Gastrointestinal and Liver Physiology.*

More serotonin = less appetite . . . and less depression, insomnia, and migraines? In 2001, researchers from the Department of Pharmacy Sciences at Creighton University in Nebraska investigated whether HCA affected serotonin, a brain chemical linked to calmer moods, better sleep, less impulsive behavior, and decreased pain levels. Their theory: that an increase in serotonin might be behind the reduction of food intake seen in animals and humans taking HCA. They added HCA to the brain cortex of experimental animals. And, sure enough, levels of serotonin increased.

In 2002, those same researchers—led by Sunny E. Ohia, PhD, currently a professor of pharmacy at the University of Houston College of Pharmacy—once again looked at HCA and serotonin. They found that HCA prevented the "uptake" of serotonin, thereby increasing its availability to brain cells—in fact, that HCA seemed to work in the brain much the same way as the medications known as SSRIs (selective serotonin reuptake inhibitors), like Prozac, Paxil, and other antidepressant and anti-anxiety drugs. The researchers also found that HCA *decreases* levels of neuropeptide Y, a brain chemical known to stimulate appetite.

HCA, they conclude, "may prove beneficial in controlling appetite, as well as [in] the treatment of depression, insomnia, migraine headaches, and other serotonin-deficient conditions."

Along these same lines, it's interesting to note that researchers at the

Ohio State University Medical Center found that experimental animals given HCA-SX had an increased activation of the genes that control serotonin receptors in the brain. Their research was published in the journal *Gene Expression* in 2004.

"My research and other studies provide scientific evidence that using an HCA supplement may help induce weight loss," Dr. Ohia told us. "I think it is worth trying."

Exercise extra. Athletes and everyday exercisers are always looking for an edge—something to help them go a little (or a lot) longer, faster, stronger. Supplements or foods that boost athletic and exercise performance are called *ergogenics aids.* (*Ergon* is Greek for "work," or "muscle power.") HCA may be one of those aids, perhaps by "sparing" carbohydrates and thereby helping the body burn more fat for fuel.

In a study published in the *Journal of Nutritional Science and Vitaminology* in 2002, Korean researchers gave HCA to one group of athletes for five days, while another group didn't get the supplement. On each of the five days, the athletes were asked to pedal an exercise bike at a moderate pace for an hour, and then to cycle to "exhaustion"—to pedal as fast as they could until they couldn't pedal anymore. Those taking HCA pedaled longer to exhaustion. The scientists also found that those taking HCA burned more fat and fewer carbohydrates (thereby improving endurance) and had a lower respiratory exchange ratio (RER), producing less carbon dioxide (and therefore breathing more efficiently).

"HCA," conclude the researchers, "enhances endurance performance." That's in well-trained athletes. What about everyday exercisers?

In a study from Japan, published in the journal *Bioscience, Biotechnology, and Biochemistry* in 2003, researchers gave six "untrained" men (non-exercisers) HCA or a placebo for five days and then put them on exercise bikes, using the same protocol as the Korean researchers. Like the athletes, the untrained men who took HCA burned more fat and had improved RER.

In another study from Korea, published in the *Journal of Nutritional Science and Vitaminology* in 2003, untrained women who took HCA could exercise longer to exhaustion.

These results don't mean that you can take HCA and go out and win a marathon in the next Olympics. But they do mean that you might have a more comfortable experience on the treadmill, exercise bike, or stair stepper—thereby helping you stick with your exercise routine, burn more calories, and lose more weight.

HCA NAYSAYERS

Science is a little bit like politics and religion—there's a lot of disagreement over basic issues. Some scientific studies show HCA *doesn't* work to trigger weight loss or reduce appetite.

One such study appeared in 1998 in a prestigious journal: the *Journal of the American Medical Association* (*JAMA*). Scientists from the Obesity Research Center at Columbia University gave HCA or a placebo for twelve weeks to 135 overweight men and women who were on a high-fiber, low-calorie diet. The placebo group lost an average of 9 pounds; the HCA group, 7 pounds.

Their study, conclude the authors, "failed to support the hypothesis that hydroxycitric acid . . . promotes either additional weight or fat loss beyond that observed with a placebo."

Immediately, several researchers wrote to *JAMA* saying this study just didn't hold up. They pointed out that:

Calorie restriction was probably too tight. The Columbia researchers used a 1,200-calorie diet. But, as we explained earlier, HCA may work by controlling appetite and by inhibiting the formation of fat from excess carbohydrates. A very-low-calorie diet—a highly restrictive, difficult-to-follow diet—is not ideal for losing extra weight with HCA. As one researcher wrote: "The study design eliminated any opportunity to demonstrate that

HCA affects appetite, reduces food intake and inhibits fat synthesis in an unrestricted diet."

In Dr. Preuss's studies, participants ate 2,000 calories a day—a moderate rather than extreme restriction. In other words, the folks who should use HCA are *not* those who are on a severely restricted, very-low-calorie diet, but those who are watching their calories a little bit, and want some extra help shedding pounds. And that's most of us.

The level of HCA was probably too low. Compared to the studies conducted by Dr. Preuss and his colleagues, the Columbia researchers may have used a low level of HCA, which probably played a role in their lack of positive findings. (We say "may have" because the researchers didn't report the level of HCA they used.)

The form of HCA was probably not ideal. The Columbia researchers used a form of HCA that is not as well absorbed, or "bioavailable," as HCA-SX. As a researcher from Italy wrote, "The bioavailability of the HCA product tested was not known—a quality factor that might significantly affect the results, because many HCA products available on the market today have low bioavailability."

HOW TO USE HCA

The key to taking HCA effectively is: use the right form, at the right time, in the right amount.

Use the most absorbable form of HCA. The two studies Dr. Preuss helped conduct were done with a form of HCA called HCA-SX (Super CitriMax), an ingredient formulated by the company Interhealth and used in HCA-containing supplements distributed by other companies. HCA-SX combines HCA with calcium and potassium, creating a biochemical that is efficiently dissolved—and therefore *maximally* absorbed from the gut and into the bloodstream and cells. Many HCA products, however, are only combined with calcium. Those products are *not* efficiently dissolved—and are therefore poorly absorbed, or not as bioavailable.

Take it three times a day, right before a meal. Studies in laboratory animals show that HCA is best absorbed on an empty stomach. In the study by Dr. Preuss and his colleagues, the participants took their HCA three times a day, thirty minutes *before* breakfast, lunch, and dinner. And taking HCA right before a meal has advantages beyond better absorption.

HCA helps stop you from feeling hungry: if you take it right before a meal, you're likely to eat less, without feeling deprived.

HCA reduces the formation of fat from carbohydrates in food: if you take it right before a meal, it has a better chance of stopping carbs from turning into fat.

Take a sufficient dose. In many studies—and in many products on the market—the dose of HCA is too low to produce a positive effect. Extrapolating from studies conducted on laboratory animals, Dr. Preuss and his colleagues determined that the ideal dose for weight loss was likely to be 2,800 milligrams (mg) a day of HCA. HCA-SX is 60 percent HCA. So, to deliver 2,800 mg of HCA a day, they gave the participants 4,667 mg of HCA-SX, in divided doses of 1,555 mg. For maximum effectiveness, Dr. Preuss recommends a similar dose: 4,500 of HCA-SX a day, in three divided doses of 1,500 mg each. He thinks the *minimum* effective dose is 1,500 mg of HCA, delivered in three 500 mg doses. To get that, you'll need to take 2,100 mg of HCA-SX—700 mg, three times a day. (Other forms of HCA may require higher or lower doses.)

CHOOSING A PRODUCT

The product on the market that Dr. Preuss's studies show is effective is HCA-SX, or Super CitriMax. For a list of supplements on the market con-

SUPPLEMENT SUPPORTER

JULIA GRIGGS HAVEY
www.juliahavey.com

Author, *Awaken the Diet Within* and *The Vice-Busting Diet*; Master Motivator, eDiets.com

She added 65 pounds during her first pregnancy. Fifty more in the next one. And, she says, "20 more pounds with no such excuse." For ten years she was more than 100 pounds overweight. And then Julia Griggs Havey lost 130 pounds, won the Mrs. Missouri beauty contest, self-published a self-help book about her life and weight-loss success, which was picked up and republished by Warner Books, and today is an internationally recognized self-help expert in losing weight. Her winning philosophy?

"Each person who is overweight has a couple of habits that are the biggest contributors to their excess weight," she told us. "They need to start working on these—one at a time. Is it the trip to the candy machine at lunch hour? The fact that there's *no* exercise in your life? Slow, gradual changes in these habits—not the steep slope of strict menus and new eating plans—are what is going to make the real difference in permanent weight loss."

In that context, she says, weight-loss supplements can have a role. "Supplements can be used as a tool to complement healthy choices, healthy actions, and healthy living." Julia says that many of the overweight women she talks to have good things to say about their experience with HCA.

"But it's like driving a car—first you need to put in the gasoline, and *then* an additive can improve function. A supplement is the additive."

taining Super CitriMax in adequate doses, please see the Web site www.supercitrimax-cs.com.

HCA plus chromium: a combination punch against pounds. In another chapter in this book, we discuss niacin-bound chromium (ChromeMate), a form of the mineral that can help weight loss by regulating blood sugar levels. In his studies on HCA, Dr. Preuss tested three groups: a placebo group; an HCA group; and a group who got HCA *and* niacin-bound chromium. The HCA-chromium group did even *better* in losing weight than those getting HCA alone. For example, in the study on sixty people, the placebo group lost an average of 3½ pounds, the HCA-SX group 10 pounds—but the HCA *and* chromium group lost 12½ pounds.

Some products with both HCA-SX and niacin-bound chromium in them include: Super CitriMax plus ChromeMate from Molecular Biologics; Super CitriMax from Now Foods; and Weight Loss Support from YouthFlow.

SAFE—FOR THOUSANDS OF YEARS

It's not enough for a weight-loss supplement to be effective. It has to be *safe*. You have to feel confident that you can take it every day without worrying about your health. HCA has a proven safety record.

It's already in the diet. HCA has been a component of the diet in southern India and Sri Lanka for thousands of years, used in curing fish, in the preparation of curries, and in many other traditional recipes.

It doesn't cause side effects in clinical studies—or in everyday use. No one dropped out of Dr. Preuss's studies because of suffering significant side effects from taking HCA-SX. And HCA has been on the market for a decade without any reports of significant ill effects.

Massive doses aren't toxic to animals. In a study published in *Molecular and Cellular Biochemistry* in 2002, experimental animals were given massive doses of HCA-SX—with no toxic or damaging results. "HCA-SX is a safe, natural supplement," conclude the authors.

That's the kind of proof—a history of safe use in food and as a dietary supplement; no side effects in medical studies; no toxic effects when massive doses are given to animals—that scientists use to declare a substance is safe. HCA is one of those substances.

However, as with any supplement or medication, pregnant and lactating women should not use HCA, nor should growing children. And you should take HCA or any supplement only with the approval and under the supervision of a doctor.

That advice goes double for people with high blood pressure or diabetes. HCA can help lower blood pressure and blood sugar levels, possibly making your current dose of antihypertensive or antidiabetic medication too high.

4

The Fat That Keeps You Thin

- MCT (Medium-Chain Triglycerides)

Just about anybody can *lose* weight. And if you're like many Americans, you've probably proven that fact to yourself—more than once!

You went on a diet. You shed the pounds you wanted to shed. You felt happy and proud. And then—slowly but oh so surely—you watched those pounds return. And maybe you went out and bought the next diet book to hit the bestseller list, diligently following its recommendations—only to find yourself repeating the same cycle of loss, gain . . . and *utter* frustration. Yo-yo you.

Yes, the hard part about losing weight is *keeping* it off. Four out of five people who shed pounds on a weight-loss program gain them all back—calorie by calorie and pound by pound, day by day and year by year. How discouraging!

Well, what if there was a nutritional supplement that "tricked" your metabolism into burning just enough extra calories every day so that those pounds *didn't* come creeping back? What if there was a supplement containing a natural substance that studies conducted by world-class nutritionists showed could help incinerate diet-busting calories?

Since you're reading this book, you've probably guessed what we're about to say next: there *is* such a supplement. But here's a fact that may take you by surprise: the primary ingredient in this supplement is a *fat*—an unusual type of fat called a *medium-chain triglyceride*. A *fat* might help keep you *thin*? Read on . . .

CLARIFYING FAT

Confused about fat? You're not alone. For decades, experts said that eating a diet low in fat was the key to a slimmer, healthier you. But even though we cut our collective fat intake—from 40 percent of the calories in our diet in the 1970s, to 33 percent today—we didn't get any thinner. Just the opposite. Over the past couple of decades, Americans (and the rest of the world) have gotten a whole lot fatter, with more than two out of three citizens now officially classified as overweight. We obeyed the experts, we ate less fat—and we got fatter. Huh?

Now, combine that mystifying trend with the nutritional reality that there are more *types* of fat than you can shake a French fry at. There's . . .

Saturated, found mostly in meat and dairy products. *Monounsaturated*, in foods like olive oil, canola oil, and avocados. *Polyunsaturated*, in corn, sunflower, and other vegetable oils. *Trans fat*, in many baked goods. *Omega-3*, in fish. And then there's *cholesterol*, the fat in your blood.

Well, relax. Fat isn't as complex as it seems.

When you understand that there's no such thing as a "bad" fat or a "good" fat (ideas based mainly on profit and politics); when you understand that fats are not nutritional devils, but a natural part of a healthy daily diet; when you look for the truth in systematic scientific results rather than sudden sensational claims—then you can easily understand and apply the facts about fat.

So let's take a closer look at fat—a *much* closer look.

Fat Under a Microscope

Put a tiny glob of fat or drop of oil under a super-powerful microscope that displays the bricks of atoms and the buildings of molecules, and you'll see *triglycerides*, the basic chemical component of fat.

Triglycerides are true to their name: they consist of three (tri) fatty acids hooked up to glycerol, a type of molecule scientists label an *alcohol*.

Those fatty acids are *chains*—the links are carbon atoms, with lots of dangling hydrogen and some baubles of oxygen. The chains vary in length. Some are short, with four to six carbon atoms. Some are long, with up to twenty-four carbon atoms.

Medium-chain triglycerides (MCT) are more like a bracelet than a necklace: they have eight to twelve carbon atoms. And because of their length, the body digests them very differently than other fats.

DIGESTING MCT:
A CALORIE-BURNING CHAIN OF EVENTS

Before telling you more about the digestion of MCT, we'd like to introduce you to two nutritional scientists who have conducted a lot of research on MCT and weight loss: Marie-Pierre St-Onge, PhD, an assistant professor in the Department of Nutrition Sciences at the University of Alabama in Birmingham, and Peter J. H. Jones, PhD, professor of Food Science and Human Nutritional Sciences at the University of Manitoba, in Canada. We interviewed them to get the most up-to-date information, insights, and practical advice about MCTs.

Long-chain triglycerides (LCTs) comprise about 90 percent of all fats, explains Dr. St-Onge. Which means that pretty much anything you eat that contains fat—tenderloin or tuna, milk or margarine, olives or Oreos—contains LCTs.

To digest LCTs, the body deposits them in "transport molecules" called *chylomicrons*: the LCTs are like passengers in the chylomicron cars. This process makes the fats *water soluble* so they can travel in the blood's liquid environment and gain entrance to watery cells. Once the LCTs buckle up, they go on a tour of your body, traveling throughout the bloodstream—until they meet up with some *hormone-sensitive lipase*, a hormone that helps deposit fat molecules in fat cells, or *adipose tissue*. At that point, it's not a tour for LCTs—it's Home Fat Home.

To recap: you eat LCTs in a food; it hitches a ride to a fat cell on a chylomicron; a hormone helps it get settled—and the next thing you know, there's a little bit more storage on your belly, butt, or thighs.

MCTs are way too cool to treat you like that.

Subtracting 100 Calories a Day—While Doing Hardly Anything!

Because of its shorter chain length, MCT doesn't need a chylomicron to get around. Instead of floating through the bloodstream and interacting with hormone-sensitive lipase, it goes straight from the stomach to the *portal circulation*—the veins and arteries that feed and drain the liver—and then to the liver itself. Dr. Jones explains what happens next:

"The liver is like a hungry blast furnace. When MCT comes rolling in directly from the gut—instead of doing that long detour around the body—it enters the furnace and increases the intensity of the flame." That means, he says, MCT increases the *energy* (calories) being *expended* by your body, an action scientists abbreviate as EE.

Yes, you heard Dr. Jones right: Digesting MCT burns extra calories! Studies show that people who get lots of dietary MCT burn an average of *100 extra calories a day* compared to people getting most of their fat as LCT.

Let's do the math: 100 calories a day equals 3,000 calories a month; 3,000 calories equals one pound of fat. Therefore, getting plenty of MCT could help prevent a weight gain of one pound per month.

That's a fat you could learn to love. So where has MCT been all your life?

THE COCONUT CONNECTION

All foods are *mixtures* of different types of fats. Dairy foods, for example, are often said to contain "saturated" fat. But the truth is, while a pat of butter contains *mostly* saturated fat, it also delivers plenty of polyunsaturated. Just so, the richest source of MCT isn't pure MCT, but it does deliver the highest level per ounce of food in nature. And the winner is . . . coconut oil.

SATURATED

A Term Only a Scientist Could Love

Saturated, says Webster's, means something is "full of" something else. So maybe you thought that when they said meat and dairy products contain "saturated" fat they meant those foods were full of fat. If only it were that simple.

Saturated and *unsaturated* are science-speak. They are technical terms used to enumerate the pairs of electrons that "bond" carbon atoms in a fatty acid chain.

If one pair of electrons is shared—a single bond—the fat is *saturated*. There's no room for more electrons. If two pairs of electrons are shared—a double bond—the fat is *unsaturated*. Another electron could come along and claim a space.

If there is one double bond, the fat is *monounsaturated*. If there are several double bonds, the fat is *polyunsaturated*.

But you don't need a microscope to notice the real-world result of these molecular realities. A single bond is stable. So a food rich in saturated fat (like lard) stays pretty much the same all the time—it's always hard at room temperature. A more unstable monounsaturated fat is liquid at room temperature and solid when refrigerated. An even more unstable polyunsaturated fat (like vegetable oil) is always liquid.

Saturated with information about saturation? We'll let you get back to the chapter . . .

(Other decent but not outstanding sources of MCT include butter and palm kernel oil.)

For many years, coconut oil and palm kernel oil—the so-called "tropical" oils—got the same bad rap as meat and dairy. They were full of saturated fat, so they were bad for your heart, so you should reduce your intake, favoring polyunsaturated fat. But in the face of those anti-coconut assertions there's an undeniable fact, says Dr. Jones: "A lot of cultures in southeast Asia consume a huge amount of tropical oils and are very healthy."

That, he says, is probably because they're consuming the oils in the context of a well-balanced diet: not too much fat, not too much protein, not too many carbohydrates. Or, as that nutritional expert Dr. Goldilocks so famously declared as she ate her porridge: Just right. (We present such a well-balanced diet in Chapter 14, Step Right Up to Weight Control.)

Does that mean you should start adding lots of coconut oil to your diet? Is that the best way to get MCT?

Several books on the market tell you to do exactly that: go nuts about coconut in order to lose weight. They advise you to eat coconut cookies and coconut beef soup and coconut chicken salad and . . . well, you get the idea. Why isn't that our recommendation? For a couple of reasons.

Based on the results of their studies, Dr. St-Onge and Dr. Jones recommend MCT not as an aid for weight loss but as an aid for *weight maintenance*. Its proven power, they say, is to *prevent* weight gain if you're not overweight, or to *maintain* your new weight after a successful diet. (Later in this chapter, we'll tell you the practical details about using MCT to prevent weight gain.)

And Dr. Jones points out that it might be counterproductive to eat the large amount of coconut oil necessary to get enough MCT to burn a lot of calories—because eating that much saturated fat could raise cholesterol levels, harming your heart.

Also, many of the scientific studies showing MCT may help burn more calories, decrease body fat, reduce hunger, and maintain weight loss used not coconut oil but a special oil that included MCT *and* several cholesterol-lowering factors.

And that special oil is now available as a nutritional supplement.

We'd like you to look at a few of those studies in detail—because if you're thoroughly convinced by the scientific evidence that MCT works, you'll be thoroughly motivated to use it to maintain weight loss.

A PEDIGREE OF SCIENTIFIC PROOF

As with most important scientific findings in the field of nutrition, the first research on MCT was done not on human beings but on animals. In the late 1980s and early 1990s, several studies showed that when animals were fed equivalent amounts of either MCT or LCT, those getting MCT had the bigger increase in EE—in other words, they burned a whole lot more calories. Scientists also conducted so-called "satiety" studies that showed animals fed MCT ate less than those receiving LCT, indicating MCT might help control appetite. Other studies showed growing animals getting MCT didn't develop as much fat as those getting LCT.

All these positive findings led scientists in the mid-1990s to begin conducting experiments on humans, measuring EE over the course of a day. Sure enough, results showed that people fed MCT burned more calories than people fed LCT. And the more MCT they got, the more calories they burned.

In an experiment by researchers in Europe, published in the *European Journal of Clinical Nutrition* in 1996, people fed 5 grams of MCT burned 10 more calories over the course of a day than people fed the same amount of LCT—while people fed 15 grams burned 32 more calories, and people fed 30 grams burned 63 more.

These and similar studies were "intriguing," as scientists like to say. But none of them showed what might happen if people got more MCT not only over the course of a day or a week, but over several weeks. Would all that extra calorie burning translate into fat loss or weight loss?

A Month of MCT

To find out, Dr. Jones, Dr. St-Onge, and other researchers conducted two studies in which they gave either MCT or LCT for twenty-eight days to overweight but otherwise healthy men and women. Then they carefully measured several factors, including weight and body fat. The studies—one on men and one on women—occurred between 1999 and 2002, when both researchers were at the School of Dietetics and Human Nutrition at McGill University in Canada. Results were published in 2002 and 2003 in the scientific journals *Obesity Research*, the *International Journal of Obesity*, and the *Journal of Nutrition*. Here's how the studies worked:

The people being studied agreed to lead strange lives for a couple of months. They ate two of their daily meals at the Clinical Nutrition Research Unit at McGill University: every breakfast, and either lunch or dinner, with the third meal prepackaged. In other words, they didn't spend *any* time during the months of the study standing in front of an open refrigerator door wondering what to have for dinner or ordering from a menu at the local restaurant. *All* of their food was prepared for them, with ingredients and portions carefully controlled, down to the last dollop of salad dressing. What were these "subjects" (as scientists call participants in a study) eating?

A diet loaded with either MCT or LCT. The MCT was part of the special formula we told you about a bit earlier: a combination of MCT oil, flaxseed oil, canola oil, and coconut oil. The LCT was in the form of either beef fat or olive oil. For the first twenty-eight days, the subjects stayed on either the MCT or the LCT diet. For the second twenty-eight days, they weren't on either diet, but the researchers continued to carefully dole out their food so that the subjects didn't gain any weight. For the third twenty-eight days, the subjects switched to the high-fat diet they weren't on during the first month—LCT subjects switched to MCT, and vice versa. At various points during both the high-MCT and high-LCT diets, the researchers took a number of different measurements.

Energy expenditure. They used highly sophisticated equipment—a so-called "metabolic monitor"—to measure the exact amount of fat and carbohydrate calories the subjects burned right after breakfast and throughout the morning. That's an important measurement since, as we've explained, the scientific theory is that MCT affects weight by being immediately processed by the liver—*no* (or very few) MCT calories are stored as fat; and *extra* calories are burned up during digestion. The researchers also calculated the average number of calories burned every day by the subjects.

Body fat. They used MRI (magnetic resonance imaging, the same technique used to detect heart disease, cancer, and other health problems) to create an extremely accurate picture of the amount of fat throughout each subject's body; each time an MRI was performed on a subject, forty-five separate images of the fat in the body were produced. (We don't think anybody kept a scrapbook.)

Body weight. They used scales, with the subjects weighing themselves every morning.

Appetite. In the study on men, five guys didn't have their meals predetermined on some of the days the scientists measured EE. Instead, they were given their standard high-MCT or high-LCT breakfast and then allowed to eat as much as they wanted at lunch, eating until they felt full. The scientists gave these five men a questionnaire about appetite and also measured the amount of food they ate at lunch.

The overall results of the studies? First, we'll tell you about the study on men and then the study on women. Because when it comes to MCT, it turns out that all subjects are not created equal.

Good News, Guys: MCT Is a Gut Buster

The men took to MCT.

More weight lost. While on MCT, the men lost an average of 2.3 pounds. While on LCT, they lost 1.4.

More fat lost. While on MCT, the men lost a lot more fat than while on LCT: the MCT diet caused them to lose 2 pounds of fat, while they lost about 7 tenths of a pound on LCT.

More gut lost. And while on MCT, the guys lost fat from where guys want to lose it the most: the gut. (Or the "Molson muscle," as Dr. Jones humorously commented, referring to the Canadian beer.) While on MCT, the men lost 1.5 pounds of upper body fat. While on LCT, they didn't lose any upper body fat.

More fat burned. While on MCT, the men burned a lot more fat after breakfast than while on LCT—about 16 percent more.

More calories burned. And men on MCT burned a lot more calories every day than men on LCT—on average, 119 more.

More appetite control. On the days tested, men getting MCT ate 221 fewer calories at lunch compared to LCT men—showing that MCT helps reduce appetite.

MCT: A Great Way to *Prevent* Weight Gain

But here's perhaps the most interesting positive finding from the study. All the men in the study were overweight. *But those who started the study with the lowest weight burned the most fat and calories while getting MCT.*

To say it plainly: the fatter guys didn't do as well on MCT. Why not? The researchers don't know for sure. But they theorize that like attracts like: the more fat cells you have, the easier it is for your body to store fat rather than burn it. Which means, they say, that MCT may be far more effective as a way to *prevent* weight gain than to lose weight.

"Our studies show that MCT is unlikely to promote rapid weight loss," says Dr. St-Onge. But, she adds, "If you have lost weight, MCT may be beneficial in helping you maintain your new weight, in the context of a healthful diet."

And maintaining your post-diet weight isn't the only special skill of MCT. If you're not overweight, MCT can help you *stay* that way.

Yes, says Dr. St-Onge, Americans are putting on the pounds. But if you measured the *rate* of daily weight gain, you'd have to do it in ounces. It's very small—so small, in fact, that the extra calories burned off by getting plenty of MCT in your daily diet could possibly *prevent* that gradual addition of extra pounds.

Dr. Jones agrees: "MCT is a good strategy for maintaining weight rather than losing weight," he says. "It can tip the energetic balance between 'calories in' and 'calories out' so that your body doesn't accumulate fat."

For Women: Positive and Promising Trends

In women, that strategy may not be quite as effective.

"MCT raises the metabolism in men so that they burn 30 to 40 more calories per meal," says Dr. Jones. "Our study showed that women burn only 10 to 15."

The study also showed that women didn't lose more weight or fat on MCT as compared to LCT. But don't give up on MCT just because you've got two X chromosomes. The study on women showed a real, measurable boost in calorie burning with MCT—so much so, says Dr. St-Onge, that if the study had gone on for a few more months it probably would have shown MCT-caused fat burning and weight loss.

Why is MCT more effective in men than in women? It could be hormones. It could be other factors. At this point, the researchers simply don't know.

MCT SUPPLEMENTS: THE HEALTHFUL OPTION

In the April 2004 issue of the *American Journal of Clinical Nutrition*, scientists from Denmark reported a study in which they gave seventeen healthy, young men diets rich in either MCT or LCT for twenty-one days. At the beginning and end of the study, these scientists measured blood fats—the fats that can clog arteries, increasing your risk of a heart attack or stroke. (Remember, MCT is a saturated fat, which scientists have said for decades can harm your arteries.)

The Scandinavian scientists measured: total cholesterol; LDL cholesterol (the "bad" kind that helps deposit fat in the arteries); the ratio of LDL to HDL cholesterol (the "good" kind that carts fat to the liver for disposal); blood triglycerides (another marker of arterial disease); and plasma glucose,

MONOLAURIN

MCT with Extra Bio-Oomph

As we said in the main part of this chapter, MCT is a *class* of fatty acids, just like horses are a class of mammals. There are many breeds of horses. And there are several kinds of MCT.

The most common are caproic acid, caprylic acid, capric acid, myristic acid, and lauric acid. And the last in that list is definitely not the least.

Lauric acid is the main antiviral and antibacterial substance in mother's milk. In the body, it changes into the biochemical *monolaurin*. And monolaurin is monomaniacal about microbes—it can hunt them down and kill them, whether they be bacteria, viruses, or fungi.

In an animal experiment conducted by Dr. Preuss, monolaurin was very effective in killing *Staphylococcus aureus*, the bacteria that usually causes food poisoning. All laboratory animals infected with the bacteria died within seven days. But in a group of staph-infected animals that were given monolaurin, half of the group survived for thirty days. Monolaurin also took down *H. pylori*, the bacteria responsible for ulcers. This research was published in *Toxicology Mechanisms and Models*, in 2005.

In the future, a natural antibiotic like monolaurin could play a crucial role in the treatment of infectious diseases—because the overuse of antibiotics has rendered many of these once-powerful drugs ineffective, as wily germs like staphylococci and tuberculosis mutate into strains that are *antibiotic-resistant*. Or a doctor might recommend you take monolaurin to prevent an infection.

Monolaurin supplements are widely available, but Dr. Preuss does not recommend self-treatment for preventing or treating infections. If you take monolaurin, do so with the recommendation and under the supervision of a doctor or other qualified health professional.

or blood sugar (high levels increase the risk for diabetes, a disease that damages circulation and often leads to heart attack and stroke).

And, sure enough, the guys getting MCT scored a lot worse than the guys getting LCT. They had: 11 percent higher total cholesterol; a 12 percent higher ratio of LDL to HDL; 22 percent higher blood triglycerides—and higher glucose.

Beware of extra MCT—you'll stay thin . . . but die of a heart attack!

Is that the moral of this scientific story?

Not if you get the right kind of MCT.

Lipid-Lowering MCT

In their studies, professors St-Onge and Jones used an oil that was not only rich in MCT, but also flaxseed and phytosterols. Why these two other ingredients?

Flaxseed oil contains a type of fatty acid called *omega-3* (also found in fish oil) that many studies show may help prevent heart disease. (And many other conditions. Omega-3 fatty acids cause the body to generate hormones that are anti-inflammatory—and inflammation is now widely recognized as a definite or possible factor in a range of diseases, including Alzheimer's, autoimmune diseases like rheumatoid arthritis, and some cancers.)

Phytosterols are a class of cholesterol-like substances in plants that actually *lower* cholesterol in the body. (Which is why oats and oat bran, for example, are so good for your heart: they're particularly rich in *beta-glucan*, one type of cholesterol-lowering phytosterol.)

But Dr. St-Onge and Dr. Jones don't just *think* the high-MCT oil they devised is good for your heart. They've proved it.

High MCT—But Low Cholesterol

Okay, now it's time to tell you: our two researchers also looked at blood fats when they did their studies on MCT. Their study on men and blood fats appeared in the June 2003 issue of the *Journal of Nutrition*. In men getting the special MCT-rich oil, total cholesterol decreased by 12.5 percent and LDL cholesterol decreased 13.9 percent. Their conclusion: the version of MCT oil used in their studies can actually *lower* the risk of heart disease and stroke in men.

Their study on women appeared in the June 2003 issue of *Metabolism*.

In women getting the special MCT-rich oil, total cholesterol decreased 9.1 percent more than it did in women getting LCT. And LDL decreased by 16 percent more on MCT than LCT. The researchers concluded that consuming an oil rich in MCT, omega-3 fatty acids, and phytosterols "improves the overall cardiovascular risk profile of overweight women."

A Source for Healthy MCT Oil

So where can you get this special, cholesterol-lowering MCT oil? Check out the Web site of Nutritional Fundamentals for Health at www.nfh.ca. This is the site of an organization of top Canadian doctors and nutritional scientists who are, says Dr. Jones, creating "evidence-based, quality-assured, toxin-free" supplements for health professionals to give to their patients—supplements that scientific studies have proved work to improve health, in one way or another. (And that's one of the main measures we use throughout *The Natural Fat-Loss Pharmacy* as we evaluate supplements: has it been *proven* to work? If it hasn't, why bother taking it?) The oil is sold there under the brand name Slim Smart.

It contains MCT and plant sterols but *not* omega-3 fatty acids, the third ingredient in the oil used in Dr. Jones's study. To get the omega-3s, you'll need to take an omega-3 supplement, and one is sold at the site: Trident SAP 3:2. "Slim Smart should be used in combination with 1 gram of omega-3 fish oils, such as Trident SAP 3:2," counsel the doctors who run the site. "The synergistic [combined] effects of Slim Smart and Trident SAP 3:2 provide overall benefits in maintenance of ideal lean body weight."

If you're interested in taking this MCT oil in supplement form (along with omega-3), talk to your doctor, and determine whether MCT is right for you as part of a total program of weight maintenance. If it is, your physician can order these products through the Web site. Follow the dosage recommendations on the labels.

PART II

Insulin Regulators

5

Shine Up Your Muscles and Pare Down Your Fat

- Chromium

The discovery of chromium as an essential nutrient—a mineral that human beings can't live without—was a matter of life and death. Literally.

The year was 1977. For the past three years, a woman with a chronic digestive condition had been receiving TPN—total parenteral nutrition, an intravenous solution that was (supposedly) supplying all of her nutritional needs. Suddenly and unexpectedly, her health took a turn for the worse.

She lost 5, 10, 20 pounds—and kept losing.

She developed severe *peripheral neuropathy*—damage to the part of the nervous system that sends information from the brain and spinal cord to the rest of the body, with symptoms like numbness, tingling, and burning in the hands and feet. Diabetics often suffer from peripheral neuropathy, so her doctors gave her a *glucose tolerance test*, which shows how the body utilizes glucose, or blood sugar. Her results were abnormal.

She was given *insulin*, the hormone that regulates blood sugar. Hardly any improvement.

She was given extra glucose. Very little improvement.

Then her doctors recalled earlier research showing that chromium can improve glucose tolerance. And because her TPN contained *no* chromium (it wasn't considered an essential nutrient at the time), they theorized a chromium deficiency might be causing her problems. Tests showed that her blood levels of chromium were abysmally low—fourteen times below normal. The doctors added chromium to her TPN.

Almost immediately, she began gaining weight. After two weeks, her glucose tolerance had normalized. After five months, her weight had normalized and her peripheral neuropathy was gone.

From then on, chromium was a permanent part of her TPN (and within the next two years or so, of everybody else's), and she never suffered from those problems again.

Chromium, concluded her doctors, is an essential nutrient—and its deficiency causes a severe disruption in blood sugar metabolism.

But we Americans aren't suffering from a chromium deficiency, right? Even for those on TPN, chromium is now part of the mix. And look at all those shiny bumpers!

Well, could the fact that 21 million Americans have type 2 diabetes, a blood sugar disorder—and that one out of four Americans is *insulin resistant*, which often sets the stage for diabetes; and that two out of three Americans are overweight, a problem that often goes hand in hand with blood sugar difficulties—have anything to do with a need for more sugar-regulating chromium in our lives?

Want to know the answer to that question? Keep reading. Because what you don't know about chromium *can* hurt you.

CHROMIUM 101

There are two kinds of chromium: the kind used for chrome plating (hexavalent chromium) and the kind your body uses to stay healthy (trivalent chromium). In the three decades since scientists discovered that trivalent chromium is an essential nutrient, they've discovered quite a few other facts about the mineral:

- *Chromium plays a key role in the regulation of your insulin system.* Hormones are chemical executives that tell cells, organs, and systems what to do. The hormone *insulin* oversees the digestion and distribution of *glucose*, or blood sugar, your body's basic fuel. Insulin helps move blood sugar out of the bloodstream and into the cells—for example, into muscle cells for instant energy, into liver cells for short-term storage, and into fat cells for layaway. Insulin does that by acting like a key, opening the lock of *insulin receptors* to let sugar in.

  Chromium helps insulin do its job, keeping blood sugar levels balanced. When chromium is on the job, blood sugar tends to go immediately into *muscle cells*, where it's used for energy. When chromium isn't on the job, blood sugar tends to float around in the bloodstream, eventually going into *fat cells* for storage.

- *You're probably not getting enough chromium in your diet.* The government's "daily value" for chromium is 120 micrograms (mcg). Most Americans get 25 to 35 in their diets. Some experts say optimal intake may be 250 mcg—or many times more.

- *Supplemental chromium—at doses four to eight times higher than the daily value—can help treat type 2 diabetes.* Studies show that 400 to 1,000 mcg a day of chromium can relieve and even reverse many of the signs and symptoms of diabetes.

- *Supplemental chromium might do more than regulate blood sugar levels—it might help you add muscle and shed fat, building a trimmer, firmer, more attractive body.* In a minute, we'll tell you about a study conducted by Dr. Preuss that showed just this result.

- *Supplemental chromium might not only help you look younger—it might also help you live longer.* Could regulation of blood sugar metabolism be a key—perhaps even *the* key—to healthy aging and longevity? And could supplemental chromium help accomplish that result? Dr. Preuss thinks so. He has published more than a dozen scientific papers on chromium, and considers it one of the most beneficial supplements for blood sugar balance, muscle gain, fat loss, and overall health.

Let's take a look at his study on chromium and dieting, published in the scientific journal *Diabetes, Obesity and Metabolism*. (It's no accident the name of that journal links diabetes and obesity. As we said a moment ago—and as you'll see throughout this chapter—blood sugar problems and over-weight often go together, a condition some researchers have dubbed "diabesity.")

WEIGHT LOSS, MUSCLE LOSS, AND THE SECRET OF SUCCESSFUL DIETING

Two people go on a diet. Before they start, both undergo DEXA, a sophis-ticated test measuring body fat and muscle mass. After four weeks, Dieter #1 has lost 6 pounds and Dieter #2 hasn't lost an ounce. Dieter #1 is the weight-loss winner, right?

Not according to a second DEXA test.

Dieter #1 lost 3 pounds of fat and 3 pounds of muscle.

Dieter #2 lost 3 pounds of fat—and gained 3 pounds of muscle.

Which dieter would you rather be: hollowed-out #1 or firmed-up #2?

Well, Dr. Preuss's study on twenty overweight African-American women shows that you can improve your chances of being like Dieter #2—if you take chromium.

African-American Women and Overweight

Dr. Preuss had a friend who managed a health club specializing in wellness for African-American women—the American women with the highest rates of overweight (78 percent), and obesity (51 percent).

(Let's pause a moment to define *overweight* and *obesity*. As used by the government, these terms indicate a particular BMI. Overweight is a BMI of 25 to 29.9. Obesity is a BMI of 30 to 39.9. Severe obesity is a BMI of 40 or higher. So, for example, a five-foot-five-inch woman weighing 150 pounds has a BMI of 25. At 180 pounds, her BMI is 30. At 220 pounds, it's 35. Now back to the study . . .)

Dr. Preuss asked the owner of the club if any of her members would like to participate in a scientific experiment testing a new, natural supplement that might help with weight loss. She put the word out and (needless to say) got twenty very eager volunteers.

As part of the study, the women were given advice on how to lower the calories in their everyday diets. And for the five months of the study, they exercised a minimum of three times a week, under the supervision of one of the study's coauthors.

Ten of the women received a placebo for two months. Then they didn't get any type of pill for one month, while they continued on their diet and exercise program. Then they switched to *niacin-bound chromium* for two months, taking 600 mcg a day. (We'll talk more about this particular form of chromium—as well as other forms, such as chromium picolinate—later in the chapter.)

From Fat to Firm

"Weeks into the study, some of the women were complaining to me that their daily trip to the scale wasn't showing any weight loss," says Dr. Preuss. "Then they'd say, 'But our dress sizes are getting smaller!' Even then, it didn't quite 'click' with me that, although the women *weren't* losing weight, they *were* gaining muscle and losing fat. But when I began to analyze the data—well, that was an eye-opener."

The ten women lost the same amount of weight while on the placebo and on chromium: 2.6 pounds on the placebo and 2.5 pounds on chromium.

While on the placebo, they lost 2.4 pounds of what scientists call *non-fat mass* (mostly muscle) and 0.2 pounds of fat.

While on chromium, they lost 2.1 pounds of fat and 0.4 pounds of non-fat mass.

In other words, the chromium group and the placebo group lost just about the same amount of weight. But:

The chromium group lost 84 percent fat and 16 percent muscle, while the placebo group lost 92 percent muscle and 8 percent fat!

"I learned that if I only looked at scale weight, chromium didn't produce results," says Dr. Preuss. "But if I looked at the relationship of muscle to fat, the women on chromium were gaining much more muscle and losing much more fat."

Lose Muscle, Regain Fat

This is not what happens to your typical dieter, who—like the women in Dr. Preuss's study who didn't get chromium—loses mostly muscle and only a little bit of fat. Unfortunately, that's exactly the wrong way to keep weight off. Here's why:

What's the more active part of your body—your tush or your triceps? Right, your triceps—muscles are naturally more active and burn more calories than fat. When you lose muscle during weight loss, you end up with a body that burns fewer calories per day. Slowly but surely, you gain your weight back . . . as fat! And because you now have a fattier, less metabolically active body, you're likely to gain back even *more* weight than you lost.

And that is exactly what happens to 90 percent of all people who lose weight, a scenario called the "yo-yo effect." You drop the weight, you gain it back, you drop the weight, you gain it back . . . talk about being toyed with!

Adding chromium to your weight-loss regimen can help *prevent* that vicious cycle, helping you gain muscle where you've got fat.

Staying Power

The group of ten women who got chromium first and the placebo second also lost more fat than muscle when they were on chromium—and *continued* to lose more fat than muscle while on the placebo!

SUPPLEMENT SUPPORTER

LINDA SPANGLE, RN, MA

www.100dayschallenge.com

Author, *100 Days of Weight Loss* and *Life Is Hard, Food Is Easy*; owner, Weight Loss for Life, a national coaching, speaking, and training program

Linda Spangle has been a weight-loss specialist for twenty years, helping thousands of people overcome their weight-loss failures. She gives dieters the insights and skills to overcome emotional eating, get control over their food (including at restaurants and social occasions), and stay motivated until they've met their goals. Ninety percent of her clients have maintained their weight loss a year after going through one of Linda's programs—compared to the average 10 percent of dieters who typically maintain their weight. And Linda thinks weight-loss supplements can be part of that success.

"During the fifteen years that I ran a weight-loss clinic I saw many people who clearly saw improvement in their weight-loss efforts by using supplements, particularly chromium and CLA," she told us. "Chromium seems to help people who are really stuck lose weight a little bit better. And I've known many dieters over the years who have used CLA as an adjunct and felt like it gave their efforts a boost."

"The chromium effect was *lasting*," says Dr. Preuss.

He'd already proven chromium's staying power during a study on laboratory animals. Rats fed high-sugar diets developed high blood pressure. When they were given chromium, their blood pressure fell. When they were taken off chromium, blood pressure *remained* low for several more weeks. (There haven't been any studies on chromium and blood pressure in humans.)

The practical impact of that finding, says Dr. Preuss, is that you can take 600 mcg of chromium for a few months to kick-start your weight-loss program, and then cut back to a maintenance dose of 200 mcg or so.

MORE PROOF OF CHROMIUM'S
FAT-BUSTING POWER

Dr. Preuss isn't the first or only scientist to show that chromium supplements can help you gain muscle and lose fat. Let's look at a couple of other studies that have helped prove the same point: chromium shines up your body's bumpers.

Twenty-eight times more muscle. Ten young men on a weightlifting program were divided into two groups, one getting chromium and the other not. After forty days, those taking the mineral had an increase in muscle of 3.5 pounds. Those getting the placebo saw an increase of . . . 2 ounces. The study was led by Gary Evans, PhD, an expert in chromium, and published in the *International Journal of Biosocial and Medical Research*.

First and ten—for muscle gain and fat loss. In a study conducted by a colleague of Dr. Evans, a group of football players either did or didn't take chromium during the six weeks of their off-season training period. Those taking chromium lost 7.5 pounds of fat and gained 5.7 pounds of muscle. Those getting a placebo lost 2.2 pounds of fat and gained 4 pounds of muscle.

Fat loss—without exercise. Led by Gil Kaats, PhD, researchers in Texas at the Health and Medical Research Foundation and the University of Texas Health Science Center conducted two studies on chromium. In one study, they gave either chromium (200 mcg or 400 mcg a day) or a placebo to 122 people. These folks weren't exercisers and they were told not to change their diets in any way. After ten weeks, the 400 mcg group had lost 4.6 pounds of fat, while the 200 mcg group lost 3.4. The placebo group lost 0.8 pounds of fat.

In another study, Dr. Kaats and his team looked at thirty women and ten men, all overweight. First, they were put on a low-fat, low-calorie diet for eight weeks. Then they were put on the same diet—with 400 mcg chromium added. At the end of the study, the participants had lost an average of about 15 pounds—with nearly 12 pounds from fat! The studies were published in *Current Therapeutic Research* in 1996 and 1998.

Losing weight—but not losing muscle. In a study published in the *International Journal of Obesity*, Austrian researchers put people on a low-calorie diet for eight weeks (800 calories a day, a highly restrictive diet that requires medical supervision). The people were divided into four groups, one of which received chromium. Everybody lost weight, of course. But only the group getting chromium didn't lose any muscle mass.

HOW CHROMIUM WORKS

Chromium works by shifting insulin from fourth into fifth gear—it boosts the hormone's sugar-handling power. How does chromium do it?

If you've been attentive to nutrition for as long as we have, you may remember reading that chromium works by helping to form the *glucose tolerance factor* (GTF), a compound purported to help insulin guide glucose into cells. GTF was an interesting theory—but it's not a reality. Truth is, scientists still aren't sure exactly how chromium works.

And it's not easy to find out. We're not talking about a hunky mineral like calcium that forms bones. We're talking about a *trace* mineral, found in your body not in the *milligrams* used to measure calcium, magnesium, iron, and zinc, but in *micrograms* (one thousandth of a milligram). How could your health be so dependent on such a tiny particle?

To answer that question, we talked to Richard Anderson, PhD, a researcher at the Beltsville Human Nutrition Research Center in Maryland, author of seventy studies on chromium, and regarded by Dr. Preuss as one of the world's leading experts on the mineral.

Dr. Anderson had us get very cozy with the insulin receptors on cells. Every cell has them, with red blood cells having as few as forty, and liver and fat cells having more than 200,000. Chromium either activates or deactivates each of two *enzymes* (proteins that trigger biochemical actions) that play key roles in how the receptor works. Chromium activates *tyrosine kinase*, which helps insulin attach to insulin receptors. It deactivates *tyrosine phosphatase*, which can block the function of insulin receptors. And chromium actually increases the number of insulin receptors.

To summarize, chromium may:

- Make more insulin receptors.

- Boost an enzyme that helps receptors work.

- Block an enzyme that turns receptors off.

Not a bad day's work for a microgram. And chromium's insulin-regulating power can not only help you build muscle and lose fat. As we mentioned earlier, it can also help prevent or reverse a disastrous disease afflicting millions of Americans: diabetes.

CHROMIUM VS. DIABETES

As this book was being written, a three-part story appeared in the *New York Times* about that city's biggest public health problem—a new and vicious epidemic. Not tuberculosis. Not AIDS. Not bird flu. No, the article was about *type 2 diabetes*, with more than one out of eight New Yorkers afflicted, and the numbers sure to rise.

The numbers aren't much better nationwide, with tens of millions of Americans suffering from the disease. And, as the article pointed out, the future looks grim too: one in three children born in the U.S. in the last five years is expected to become diabetic in his or her lifetime, perhaps lowering the average life expectancy of Americans for the first time in more than a century.

Why the epidemic in NYC and the rest of the country?

Too many calories and too much sugary, fatty food, leading to decreased insulin sensitivity, the first step in developing diabetes.

And too little chromium—which can help regulate insulin—in the diet, says Dr. Anderson.

Let's look at some of the evidence that supplemental chromium might help you prevent diabetes or control it if you have it:

Insulin sensitivity. High levels of insulin in the blood—called *hyperinsulinemia*—are the first sign of insulin resistance. Ten scientific studies have shown that supplementing the diet with chromium can help lower high insulin levels. In one study on twenty-nine overweight people with a family history of type 2 diabetes, those who took 1,000 mcg of chromium picolinate a day had improved insulin sensitivity. Those who took a placebo didn't.

Type 2 diabetes. Although some studies haven't shown a positive effect on type 2 diabetes, Dr. Anderson points out that most of them didn't use enough chromium (a minimum of 400 mcg a day) or a highly absorbable form of chromium (like chromium picolinate). "Essentially," he says, "*all* of the studies using the more bioavailable chromium picolinate have reported positive effects, with greater effects at 1,000 mcg per day compared with 200 mcg per day." He cites one study in which people with type 2 diabetes given 1,000 mg of chromium a day had significantly lower blood sugar levels after two months.

Lower cholesterol, too. He also notes that they had lower levels of cholesterol—another well-proven benefit of taking "extra" chromium.

In another study of 800 patients with type 2 diabetes, chromium supplements helped control blood sugar levels *and* many of the symptoms of type 2 diabetes, like excessive thirst and urination, and fatigue.

Type 1 diabetes. People with type 1 diabetes—the autoimmune disease that usually starts in childhood, with the body attacking and destroying the insulin-generating cells of the pancreas—may also benefit from more chromium, says Dr. Anderson. In one study of 162 patients with type 1 diabetes, people who took 200 mcg a day of chromium picolinate were able to reduce their average insulin dosage by 30 percent.

Gestational diabetes. Pregnant women are at a higher risk for developing diabetes—a disease that's not good for the mother-to-be or her developing baby. In a study, thirty women with gestational diabetes were divided into three groups and given 0, 4, or 8 mcg of chromium per kilogram of body weight, for eight weeks. The women getting the chromium had lower blood sugar levels—and the women getting the 8 mcg dosage had lower levels than those getting 4. "Chromium picolinate supplementation may be an adjunctive therapy when dietary strategies are not sufficient to achieve [normal blood sugar levels] in women with gestational diabetes," write the authors, in the *American Journal of Clinical Nutrition*.

Steroid-caused diabetes. Steroids—powerful, inflammation-reducing medications used to help control many diseases, from arthritis to allergies—can cause diabetes. Doctors in Israel, working with Dr. Anderson, found that steroids increased chromium losses from the urine by 75 percent.

When they supplemented several patients who had steroid-caused diabetes with chromium, they were able to reduce their average dosage of diabetes-controlling drugs by 50 percent. "Corticosteroid treatment increases chromium losses, and . . . steroid-induced diabetes can be reversed by chromium supplementation," wrote Dr. Anderson and his colleagues, in the journal *Diabetic Medicine*.

"If chromium was a drug, everybody would have touted it as a 'wonder drug' after the results of this study," Dr. Anderson told us. "But effective nutritional treatments almost never get that kind of positive attention."

IS AGING A CHROMIUM DEFICIENCY?

Let's leave Dr. Anderson in his Beltsville, Maryland, laboratory, get on the Beltway, and drive over to Georgetown, to Dr. Preuss's laboratory. Once there, it's not unlikely that we'll find him contemplating one of the rodents in his laboratory that has been given chromium all its life—and lived on and on, way beyond the life span of a typical Mickey or Minnie. Why has chromium kept those old rodents alive and kicking? Because, Dr. Preuss theorizes, the mineral is stopping them from developing *insulin resistance . . .*

The Many (Unhappy) Faces of Insulin Resistance

What can happen to your body when you are insulin resistant—when the hormone can't efficiently remove sugar from the blood and put it into the cells?

Metabolic mayhem.

You can get fat, particularly around the middle, as your body stores the unused sugar.

You can get "fat" on the inside, with high levels of "bad" LDL cholesterol and triglycerides (another heart-damaging blood fat), and low levels of "good" HDL cholesterol.

You can develop high blood pressure.

And, in fact, insulin resistance, overweight, high triglycerides, low HDL, and high blood pressure are now seen as a *single* set of related problems, or a *syndrome*—called metabolic syndrome, or syndrome X.

Metabolic syndrome is not some rare problem—25 percent of Americans have it! It's a recognized risk factor for type 2 diabetes, the condition in which high levels of blood sugar become near constant and metabolic mayhem turns into metabolic tragedy, with possible (and very common) "complications" like heart attack, stroke, severe nerve damage to toes, feet, and legs leading to amputation, kidney disease, and blindness.

How Insulin Resistance Develops

Insulin resistance doesn't happen overnight. When cells first start resisting insulin, the insulin-manufacturing pancreas switches into higher gear and pumps out more of the hormone, stabilizing sugar levels. Doctors call this condition *hyperinsulinemia*. After a while, however, even those higher levels of insulin don't do the job. Blood sugar stays high. Eventually, you can develop type 2 diabetes. But between the start of insulin resistance and the onset of type 2 diabetes—there's a whole lot of *aging* going on.

Glucose on the Loose

Excess glucose in the blood triggers *glycosylation*—the sugar literally sticks to cellular material and alters its structure. (And not for the better.)

Damaged DNA. It sticks to DNA and damages it—one of the fundamental signs of aging. (And a possible cause of cancer.)

Concrete collagen. It sticks to the collagen in your skin and stiffens it—an all-too-obvious outer sign of aging. (Flexible collagen is the very essence of youthful skin.)

KO'd kidneys. It sticks to your kidney cells, weakening them so that they allow more salt in your system. (This is probably the mechanism by which insulin resistance boosts blood pressure.)

More free radicals. Extra glucose even generates more free radicals, the unstable molecules that damage cells.

In short, extra glucose ages your body in all kinds of ways, not just by setting you up for type 2 diabetes.

Keeping Rats Young

It's too scientifically complex to prove conclusively that preventing or slowing insulin resistance extends life in us humans. Rats are a different story.

When scientists feed rats a calorie-restricted diet that keeps their glucose and insulin levels very low, the rats live much longer lives than their normally fed brethren.

"The ability of caloric restriction to slow many manifestations of aging and to augment life span in rats supports a prominent role for the glucose/insulin system in the process of aging," wrote Dr. Preuss, along with his colleagues, in a paper titled "Insulin Resistance: A Factor in Aging?"

CINNAMON: ANOTHER WAY TO REGULATE INSULIN RESISTANCE

As you've read this chapter on chromium, you've discovered the mineral works to help you lose fat and gain muscle by improving the functioning of *insulin*, the hormone that regulates the level of sugar (glucose) in the blood. You've read about the effectiveness of chromium *supplements*. But what about chromium-rich *foods*?

In 1990, Dr. Richard Anderson investigated the chromium content of a range of foods and spices. He also tested them to see which of them might have chromium's proven power to supercharge insulin and balance blood sugar— what he called *insulin potentiating activity*.

Among the insulin-helping standouts in food: tuna fish and peanut butter.

Among spices: cinnamon, cloves, bay leaves, and turmeric.

Since 1990, research has continued to focus on cinnamon as a way to potentiate insulin and balance blood sugar.

Bringing down blood sugar by 29 percent. The best study on cinnamon, blood sugar, and people (there have been lots of studies on rats) was conducted in 2003 by Dr. Anderson and a team of researchers in Pakistan. They divided sixty people with type 2 diabetes into two groups. One group received cinnamon for 40 days: either 1, 3, or 6 grams daily. The other group got placebos.

Everyone taking cinnamon had drops in blood glucose levels, ranging from 18 to 29 percent. They also had lower LDL cholesterol (7 to 27 percent), and total cholesterol (12 to 26 percent). There were no significant changes in the placebo groups.

These results indicate that "the inclusion of cinnamon in the diet of people with type 2 diabetes will reduce risk factors associated with diabetes and cardiovascular disease," wrote the researchers, in the December 2003 issue of *Diabetes Care*.

How does cinnamon work? Research by Dr. Anderson and scientists at Iowa State University shows that cinnamon may actually *mimic* insulin. It stimulates insulin receptors on fat cells in the same way that insulin does, allowing excess sugar to move out of the blood and into cells. Other studies from Japan show that it does the same in muscle cells.

How can you get more cinnamon in your diet? Some suggestions from cooks we know and love: Sprinkle it on hot cereals, yogurt, or applesauce . . . use it to accent sweet potatoes, winter squash, or yams . . . try it with lamb, beef stew, or chilies . . . it even goes great with grains like couscous and barley, and legumes like lentils and split peas. Try to get one-quarter to one teaspoon daily, says Dr. Anderson.

Break the Triangle

Like wrinkles, there's no getting away from some degree of insulin resistance as you age. However, you can maintain insulin resistance at relatively normal levels for your entire life. How?

Dr. Preuss says to think of insulin resistance, overweight, and aging as the three sides of a triangle. To normalize insulin resistance, or lose weight, or slow aging—you have to "break" at least one side of that triangle.

Decreasing insulin resistance can help you lose weight—and make you look and feel younger. Losing weight often lessens insulin resistance—and makes you look and feel younger. (In fact, the two keys to *preventing* weight gain—a balanced diet and regular exercise—are key to preventing insulin resistance.)

And a number of natural strategies and supplements also have been proven to maintain normal insulin metabolism, says Dr. Preuss, including: increasing the fiber in your diet; taking antioxidant nutrients like A, C, E, selenium, and zinc; including more cinnamon in your diet; or taking a chromium supplement.

And taking a chromium supplement, he says, is the most thoroughly studied and therefore probably the best of those options. But is chromium *safe?*

SAFE AND EFFECTIVE

There's no question about it: chromium is a poison and can cause cancer. Uh, did we mention we're talking about *hexavalent chromium,* the kind used in bumpers, paints, welding, and steel making? That type of chromium *is* a toxin, proven to increase the risk of cellular damage and cancer. But *trivalent chromium,* the type found in food and used in chromium supplements, is a very different kind of mineral—the *safe* kind.

Safe to ingest in food. And safe to ingest in quantities much higher than you'd find in your diet. Chromium is considered one of the *least toxic* of nutrients, says Dr. Anderson.

The *reference dose*—the dose the government says you could take every day without harm—is *350* times higher than the RDA. That's quite a big safety factor, considering the reference dose for zinc is only twice that of the RDA.

Rats fed trivalent chromium at levels *thousands* of times higher than the reference dose for humans (based on body weight) didn't show any toxic effects.

And none of the hundreds of studies on chromium in people have shown adverse affects.

Questions About Chromium

It's not that there haven't been *any* questions about chromium, of course.

In 1995, scientists added high levels of chromium picolinate (the most commonly marketed form) to a culture of hamster ovary cells, and there were signs of chromosomal damage—signs not seen with other types of chromium, like chromium chloride and chromium poly-nicotinate.

In a more recent study, fruit flies getting massive doses of chromium picolinate had poorly formed wings.

And in the late nineties, there were two cases of people who took chromium picolinate for weight loss and developed kidney failure. One woman took 1,200 mcg to 2,400 mcg a day for four months, and the other took 600 mcg a day for six weeks.

These cases are the "exception to the rule"—*millions* of people have taken chromium supplements without harm. In fact, says Dr. Preuss, there's no absolute certainty that either case was caused by intake of chromium pi-colinate. And there are *no* reports of adverse reactions to chromium poly-nicotinate (niacin-bound chromium).

CHOOSING A PRODUCT

Go to a shopping Web site and enter the keyword "chromium," and—once you've eliminated the "Tools and Hardware" and "Craft Supplies" selections,

SUPPLEMENT SUPPORTER

JOHN GRAY, PhD

www.marsvenus.com

Author, *The Mars and Venus Diet and Exercise Solution* and many other Mars/
Venus books

In John Gray's opinion, Mars needs more chromium.

"I am a big fan of high doses of chromium for men," he told us. That's because, he says, chromium increases levels of dopamine, a brain chemical. And
when a man's brain has more dopamine, says Dr. Gray, he experiences less
stress (which leads to more fat burning), has more energy and optimism, gets
healthy, and can lose weight quickly. He recommends 500 to 1,000 mcg per day
for men. "Most men will see results in a week."

For the sake of better brain chemistry in men and women, his program also
eliminates what he calls dietary "bad guys." (Bad *guys* . . . ? Mars takes it on
the chin again!) They include hydrogenated fat, refined sugar, wheat, and dairy
products. And he recommends foods, nutritional shakes, and supplements that
supply adequate amounts of amino acids, trace minerals, protein, B vitamins,
and omega-3 fatty acids.

and narrowed in on "Nutrition"—you'll get, oh, about 1,400 different items
to choose from.

There's chromium picolinate (the most common).

There's chromium nicotinate or polynicotinate, the chromium bound
to the B vitamin niacin, and the type used in Dr. Preuss's study, under the
trademark ChromeMate.

There's GTF chromium, a labeling throwback, since no such substance
exists.

There's chromium histidinate, a relatively new and highly absorbable
form of the nutrient.

And a couple of others.

Is any one of them better than any other, in terms of helping you protect muscle and shed fat when you're dieting? Dr. Preuss says his research and that of others favors chromium bound to nicotinate (niacin), picolinate, or histidinate. (And, as you may have read in the chapter on HCA, Dr. Preuss has conducted another study in which chromium nicotinate *combined* with HCA was particularly effective at weight loss *and* fat loss. Products with that combination of nutrients are listed on page 84.)

There's nothing wrong with taking chromium as chromium picolinate (which has proven itself in many fat-loss studies), or any of its other forms. But, says Dr. Preuss, the most prudent course is to take the supplement that appears to be the safest, and that's niacin-bound chromium.

For those trying to lose weight, he recommends 600 mcg a day of niacin-bound chromium, in three divided doses of 200 mcg.

After achieving the results you want, he recommends switching to a maintenance dose of 200 mcg a day.

When should you take that chromium? "Take chromium separately from meals or multivitamin-mineral supplements," says Dr. Anderson. "There are many factors—including starch, calcium, and iron—that can interfere with the absorption of chromium."

And there's another factor that can interfere with the effectiveness of chromium—continuing to eat a high-fat, high-sugar diet.

Not an Overnight Cure for Overweight

The problem with many weight-loss supplements isn't that they don't work—it's that they're oversold. The hype and the hoax says that taking the supplement is *the only thing you have to do* to quickly and easily lose weight. And that was just the way chromium was sometimes presented when research began to show it could help people lose fat and gain muscle, says Dr. Anderson.

"There used to be commercials saying you could go from a size 16 to a size 8 dress in a couple of weeks *just* by taking chromium," he says. But chromium *doesn't* work that way.

Chromium doesn't erase fat overnight. "Chromium works gradually and progressively—you see results not in days or weeks, but in months," he says.

And you probably won't see *any* results if you continue to eat foods rich in sugar and fat. "You can't eat a diet rich in sugar and fat and still lose fat and gain muscle," says Dr. Anderson. "Chromium may help counteract some of the negative effects of such a diet, but you won't see many benefits in terms of firming and slimming."

As we say throughout the book: weight-loss supplements are an *aid* to a balanced diet and exercise. But they can't replace them.

PART III

Carbohydrate Inhibitors

Lower Your Carbs— Without a Low-Carb Diet

Supplements That Cut Starch and Sugar Absorption

- Starch Blockers (White Kidney Bean, Wheat, Hibiscus)
- Sugar Blocker (L-arabinose)

On his father's side, Dr. Preuss's genealogy is as German as a bottle of Lowenbrau. If he were to honor his ancestors' taste buds, he'd dine on bratwurst and sauerkraut. But if you sat next to him in a restaurant, you'd think his last name was Romano. He adores pasta—any kind, from angel hair to vermicelli. And he has a particular fondness for good old spaghetti and meatballs—in portions that would make an Italian grandmother proud.

That's why his antipasto usually includes an anti-pasta. An anti-pasta pill, that is.

If he knows he's going out for a big Italian dinner, he takes along a couple of pills—a hearty dose of what scientists call *carbohydrate digestive enzyme inhibitors*, and what are popularly known as *starch blockers* (the name we'll use in the rest of the chapter).

A starch-blocker supplement prevents a portion of the carbohydrates in pasta (or any other high-carb food) from being broken down quickly and absorbed immediately. Why does Dr. Preuss take those pills? To keep extra pounds off his body and to improve his insulin system. (We'll talk more about the importance of insulin in a moment.)

Decades before the Atkins and South Beach diets became popular, it was theorized that an excessive intake of refined *carbohydrates* (the starch in breadsticks, for example, or the sugar in tiramisu) could trigger the body to manufacture excessive *fat*. That theory wasn't readily accepted by the medical community or the public. But in the last decade or so, it's become generally accepted as scientific fact.

And many scientists now think that cutting down on refined carbohydrates can do a lot more than help you get and stay trim. Limiting refined carbs may help you avoid or delay serious illnesses like adult-onset diabetes, stroke, heart disease, and cancer. It may even slow the aging process.

WHAT'S WRONG WITH CARBOHYDRATES, ANYWAY?

First, let's make a clear distinction between two types of carbohydrates: *refined* and *unrefined*. In spite of the name, it's the refined variety that doesn't behave very well in your body.

Carbohydrates are one of three major nutrients that supply your body with calories, or energy; the other two are protein and fat. As the name indicates, carbohydrates are chemically composed of carbon, hydrogen, and oxygen molecules. These molecules arrange themselves into either *simple* carbohydrates (as in fruit) or *complex* carbohydrates (as in grains). Simple carbohydrates are also called *sugars*; complex carbohydrates are also called *starches*. So where do *refined* and *unrefined* fit in? Those terms indicate what happens to carbohydrates when they enter the food supply.

Remember the song "Down by the Old Mill Stream"? It was composed in 1910, when grains were milled by a stone wheel turned by hydropower. A power plant may have replaced the stream, but the process is basically the same. During milling, a grain of wheat—sporting a nutrient-filled kernel and a coat of bran—is indecorously stripped of both. Only the *refined* portion is left.

Whole wheat becomes white flour, which becomes white bread. Corn becomes corn meal, which becomes corn chips or high-fructose corn syrup. Leafy stalks of sugar cane become white sugar, which—unbecomingly—becomes your gut, butt, and thighs.

There's nothing wrong with refined carbohydrates in and of themselves. No food is inherently "bad" or "good." But when your diet is overloaded with refined carbohydrates (and chances are it is: 98 percent of the wheat eaten by Americans is white flour, and each of us ingests an average of 135 pounds of sugar a year), your bloodstream is overloaded with blood sugar, or glucose. That's not good for your waistline. Or for the rest of your body.

The Insulin Insult

When you ingest any kind of carbohydrate, it's broken down in the intestinal tract into simple sugars, like glucose, which then enter the bloodstream. In other words, carbs are turned into fuel for the body.

But your bloodstream isn't like your car's fuel tank, with "Full" being A-okay and "Empty" being AAA. Your body prefers its glucose "just right"—between 70 and 100 mg/dl (milligrams per deciliter).

Digested too fast, however, carbs are just wrong—glucose levels skyrocket. Quick-digesting carbs have a high *glycemic index* (G.I.), a measurement of how slowly or quickly carbs turn into glucose. And, needless to say, refined carbs almost always have a higher G.I. than unrefined carbs. For example, a slice of white bread has a G.I. of 100, while a slice of whole wheat is 72—which means white bread generates approximately 50 percent more glucose than whole wheat. What does your body do with all that extra glucose?

Meet your pancreas—an L-shaped, hormone-secreting endocrine gland tucked behind your stomach. The pancreas manufactures insulin, a hormone that regulates glucose. When glucose is too high, the pancreas pumps out more insulin, which attaches itself to insulin receptors located on muscle, fat, and other cells. This in turn activates other receptors that pull glucose into the cell, normalizing blood sugar levels.

But when your daily diet is loaded with high-G.I. refined carbohydrates (white bread, corn chips, bagels, doughnuts, cookies, ice cream, and soda), so much insulin is pumped into the bloodstream that insulin receptors start to wear out. Eventually, your cells become "insulin insensitive"— they're too pooped to grab on to circulating insulin (triggering your pancreas to manufacture even *more* insulin, in an attempt to compensate for the poor insulin response). You end up suffering from a state called *hyperinsulinemia*—high levels of insulin in the blood. And because the insulin system isn't working, blood sugar levels are askew. Overall, this condition is called *insulin resistance*.

Insulin resistance doesn't have any obvious symptoms—its initial damage is undetectable, except by medical testing. But over time it can harm your body. That's bad news for the 70 to 90 *million* Americans with insulin resistance.

Insulin Resistance and Overweight

Because it's such a basic metabolic malfunction, insulin resistance can affect just about every organ and system in your body. It can weaken the immune system, damage nerves, and clog arteries. It can jack up blood pressure and shove you toward diabetes. And it can be fat's best friend.

Fast food folly. In a study published in January 2005 in the prestigious medical journal *Lancet*, American scientists traced the eating habits of more than 3,000 young adults for fifteen years. Those who ate fast food twice a week or more (I'll have the white bread and high-fructose corn syrup, please, with a side of saturated fat) were on average 10 pounds heavier and had double the rate of insulin resistance compared to those who ate fast food less than once a week.

Lose and you win. In another study—conducted by researchers in the Department of Medicine at the University of Pittsburgh, and published in the journal *Diabetes*—thirty-two overweight men and women went on a weight-loss program for four months. They lost an average of 7 pounds—and their insulin resistance decreased by 19 percent.

Dr. Preuss is often asked which comes first: insulin resistance or obesity. Like the chicken and the egg, there is no obvious answer. Overweight leads to insulin resistance, and insulin resistance can lead to overweight. But while the cause and effect may not be perfectly clear, there *is* a vicious cycle in action—and, for the sake of your health, it must be stopped.

Gaining Fat and Losing Muscle

But being insulin resistant does more than just pack on extra pounds. It sets you up to gain fat *and* lose muscle. (When looking at the dangers of insulin resistance and hyperinsulinemia, many health scientists neglect this part of the equation.) The numbers on the scale may tell you that you've gained 10 pounds in the last year. But what they're not telling you is that because you've lost muscle mass at the same time, you may have gained *more* than 10 pounds of fat! How does this happen? Scientists aren't sure, but theories abound, based on literally thousands of studies that have tried to piece together the metabolic jigsaw puzzle of insulin and overweight. Some possible causes:

Fat gain. Normally, you get rid of fat through a process called *lypolysis*—fat is broken down into smaller components called *free fatty acids*, and they are *oxidized*, or burned up. Insulin slows down lypolysis. Stated most simply: more insulin circulating in the blood means less fat breakdown—fat is literally trapped in fat cells.

Muscle loss. Insulin regulates blood levels of crucial amino acids, the building blocks of protein—and protein is what muscles are made of. For example, when blood levels of insulin are high, blood levels of leucine, a muscle-making amino acid, are low.

Additionally, insulin resistance damages the insulin receptors of muscle cells, allowing less glucose into the cells. Little by little, muscles shrivel.

Summing Up: The Carbohydrate Catastrophe

Let's assess the damage.

A diet high in refined carbohydrates—quickly digested starches and sugars—can cause insulin resistance.

Insulin resistance and obesity go hand in hand.

And not only can you get fatter. You can get flabbier, as fat accumulates and muscles shrink.

The obvious solution: Cut down on the refined carbs!

But here's what's not so obvious: What's the *best* way to do that?

IS THE LOW-CARB DIET SAFE?

Americans have been obsessed with fat in food. Over the past three decades, we were trained to read nutritional labels, zero in on the percentage of fat— particularly the saturated fat found in animal and dairy products—and turn up our collective nose at products with a high fat content. Dr. Preuss believes that at least part of today's obesity epidemic—with two out of every three Americans overweight—has its roots in this obsession. Because while we focused on fat, we forgot about the calories and the carbs that replaced it. Our meals were lower in fat, but higher in calories and refined carbohydrates. And we gained a lot of weight.

But the proverbial pendulum has swung. Americans are now obsessed with lowering carbs. And what we're finding is that *any* obsessive focus on a single macronutrient—be it fat, carbohydrate, or protein—can cause health problems.

Low-Carb Lawsuit

When we were writing this chapter, Bill Gottlieb received a press release from the Physicians Committee for Responsible Medicine, a group that strongly advocates a diet rich in unrefined carbohydrates as the best way to stay healthy and trim. The news: a judge in Florida had denied a motion to have a lawsuit against the Atkins diet dismissed.

The suit had been filed by a former Atkins dieter, a fifty-three-year-old man who followed the diet for two and a half years—and developed high cholesterol, severe chest pains, and a life-threatening arterial blockage, requiring medical treatment. (His medical tests from before the diet showed no signs of heart disease.)

The dieter may or may not win his lawsuit; it may not even go to court. But the fact that there is such a lawsuit dramatically illustrates a *possible* problem with the low-carbohydrate diet: when you lower calories from carbs, you increase calories from other nutritional factors—like the potentially artery-clogging saturated fat found in the meats and dairy products that comprise a typical low-carb diet.

A raw LDL. A study conducted at Duke University, and published in the *Annals of Internal Medicine* in 2004, shows exactly what can happen. In thirteen of forty-four people on a low-carb diet for six months, levels of "bad" LDL cholesterol shot up 10 percent. In one person, LDL went from 184 to 283—tripling the risk of heart attack.

IS THE LOW-CARB DIET FUN?

Another possible problem with the low-carb diet: it's low-fun. How long can you stop yourself from eating even moderate amounts of the foods you (if you're like most people) love—the potatoes and pasta, the ice cream and cake? Not for very long.

Diet dropouts. In a study on four weight-loss diets conducted by researchers at the Tufts-New England Medical Center and published in the *Journal of the American Medical Association* in January 2005, 47 percent of the people on the Atkins diet dropped out.

And maybe a lot of other low-carb dieters are starting to do the same.

According to a report in the *New York Times*, the number of Americans on low-carbohydrate diets has dropped by nearly 50 percent.

A SMART ALTERNATIVE: CARB BLOCKERS

You've learned in this chapter that cutting down on refined carbs can help you lose weight or stay slim. But you've also learned that a low-carb diet has two possible drawbacks. Carbs might be replaced with an excess of calories, saturated fat, or trans fats. And most people can't (and don't want to) sustain a low-carb lifestyle for a lifetime.

Is there a way to cut carbs *without* going on a low-carb diet? Happily, the answer is yes.

You can block the *absorption* of refined carbohydrates in the digestive tract. You can take natural supplements that block the action of the digestive enzymes that break carbs down into absorbable sugars. These products are typically called *carb blockers*.

You heard us right: You can have your cake (at least a slice of it) and eat it too.

Two Categories of Carb Blockers

Carb blockers come in two major categories.

Starch blockers work by stopping the action of *alpha amylase*, the digestive enzyme that breaks down starch in the intestines.

Sugar blockers stop the action of *sucrase*, the digestive enzyme that breaks down sucrose, or table sugar.

Let's take a look at a few of the enzyme-arresting ingredients in carb-blocker supplements, and at the scientific studies that make a strong case for their effectiveness.

Starch Absorption That's Full of Beans

Since the 1950s scientists have known that kidney beans contain a substance that can block the action of alpha amylase in vitro, or in a test tube. In the

1970s, companies used this knowledge to develop and market starch-blocker supplements. But studies in the early 1980s in big-time journals like *Science*, the *New England Journal of Medicine*, and the *American Journal of Clinical Nutrition* showed that starch-blocker supplements didn't work in people. Oh well.

Then, in the mid-eighties, scientists figured out how to make a water-based extract of white kidney beans with extra anti-amylase activity—and an *effective* starch blocker was born.

Blockerbuster. In an experiment published in the journal *Gastroenterology* in 1986, researchers at the Mayo Clinic inserted tubes into the intestines of volunteers (paid, we hope) and measured the digestive effects of taking white bean extract. On Day 1 of the study, the volunteers took rice starch with the extract; on Day 2 they took the starch with a placebo. The extract decreased amylase activity by more than 95 percent. And (no surprise to today's carb-savvy nutritional scientists) it lowered the rise of blood sugar by 85 percent and completely eliminated increased insulin levels. In other words: it worked.

Good news for diabetics. In another study that year, published in *Mayo Clinic Proceedings*, the same researchers gave a starch blocker to diabetics and healthy people. In both groups, the starch blocker substantially reduced postmeal increases in glucose and insulin. "We conclude," wrote the researchers, that the starch blocker "is effective and potentially beneficial in the treatment of diabetes."

Fine: starch blockers can help regulate carbohydrate metabolism. But can they help you lose weight?

California Carbs

In 2004, doctors at the UCLA School of Medicine conducted an eight-week study on Phase 2, a starch blocker with white kidney bean extract as its main ingredient.

Twenty-seven overweight adults went on a low-fat, high-fiber weight-loss diet. They were divided into two groups: one group got a 1,500-milligram dose of Phase 2 at lunch and dinner, while the other got a placebo. After eight weeks, the Phase 2 group had lost twice as much weight—an average of 3.8 pounds, compared to 1.6 for the placebo group.

Another plus: levels of triglycerides (a heart-hurting blood fat boosted by refined carbohydrate intake) fell 26.3 mg/dL in the Phase 2 group, compared to an 8.2 drop in the placebo takers.

The doctors also note that the Phase 2 group had less body fat and more energy.

And nobody who took Phase 2 suffered any side effects during the study or had any negative changes in medical tests measuring liver and kidney function.

The doctors are quick to point out that their study didn't *prove* the effectiveness of carb blockers as a weight-loss aid—there were too few people enrolled in the study to supply the supercharged statistics that scientists demand before they'll declare something *proved*. But they do say their study provides an impetus to conduct more studies to try to "demonstrate conclusively" whether or not carb blockers can help you lose weight.

Well, until those conclusive studies are conducted (*if* they're ever conducted), Dr. Preuss says: Taking a starch blocker can't hurt your weight-loss efforts—and it certainly might help.

Pasta la Vista

In 2005, Leonardo Cellano, MD, a professor at the Universita Cattolica di Roma, in Rome, Italy, with the assistance of Dr. Preuss, conducted another study on Phase 2. (What better place to test a carb blocker than the Land of Pasta?)

The study participants were sixty overweight but healthy people, aged twenty-five to forty-five. For thirty days, they were given either the starch blocker or a placebo, while they were on a 2,000- to 2,200-calorie diet that included lots of carbs.

At the beginning and end of the study, the researchers took several measurements: weight; fat mass and non-fat mass (muscle); the thickness of fat tissue under the skin; and the circumference of waists, hips, and thighs.

After thirty days, those taking the carb blocker were in much better shape.

Ten times more weight loss. Those taking the starch blocker lost 6.6 pounds. The placebo group lost 6 tenths of a pound.

Losing fat, not muscle. And the pounds they were shedding weren't muscle—the carb-blocker group lost 5.3 pounds of fat mass and 1.3 pounds of non-fat mass.

Trimmer under the skin. The thickness of the fat under the skin of those taking the starch blocker decreased by 3.8 millimeters (between 1 and 2 tenths of an inch). The placebo group had a decrease of 0.6 millimeters.

Slimmer waists, hips, and thighs. The starch-blocker group lost an average of 2.8 millimeters from their waists, 1.5 from their hips, and 1.0 from their thighs. (Every little bit helps.) The placebo group had virtually no change.

Taking a starch blocker every day, even when on a carb-rich diet, can decrease body fat and maintain muscle, concluded Dr. Cellano and Dr. Preuss. And, they say, it could be an effective aid in a weight-loss or weight-maintenance program.

Wheat Works Too

Extract, extract, read all about them: a *wheat* extract can also block amylase.

Picking Slim. Researchers at the Mayo Clinic studied the carb blocker CarboSlim, which has wheat amylase inhibitor as its main ingredient. On two consecutive days of the study, twelve people (four thin, four overweight, and four overweight diabetics) either did or didn't get CarboSlim after eating breakfast. On both days, they had their glucose levels measured for seven hours after breakfast. On the day they got CarboSlim, ten of the twelve had lower glucose levels.

Hold the hunger. In a study in the journal *Nutrition*, conducted by the same researchers at the Mayo Clinic, rats getting wheat extract ate less and gained less weight than rats not getting the extract.

Allergy alert. If you're allergic to wheat, *don't* take a carb blocker with wheat extract. In an article in the *Journal of Allergy and Clinical Immunology,* researchers at the University of Arkansas identified wheat alpha-amylase inhibitor as an allergy trigger (allergen) for those who have a known allergy to wheat.

Hibiscus Extract: Tropical Carb Stopper

Hibiscus flowers are five-petaled, color-crazy blooms that cluster on tropical bushes. And they're lovely in the laboratory too: an extract of hibiscus can block carbs.

Power flower. Animal studies show that hibiscus extract inhibits the action of amylase, the digestive enzyme that breaks down carbs.

Petals to the metal. And in a 2003 study on diabetic rats, hibiscus extract cut glucose levels by up to 14 percent and insulin levels by up to 46 percent.

L-arabinose: How Sweet It Isn't

L-arabinose is itself a carbohydrate: a simple sugar found in foods like corn. Isolated, it functions as a sucrose blocker: it stops or slows the action of the digestive enzyme *sucrase*, which breaks down sugar in the intestines.

Sugar takes its lumps. A research study by Japanese scientists, published in the journal *Metabolism*, showed that L-arabinose reduced blood sugar levels in rats given a big dose of table sugar.

Facing down fat. In another Japanese study, published in the *Journal of Nutrition*, researchers again fed rats high doses of table sugar—which turned into fat. However, when the rats were fed table sugar *and* L-arabinose, fat-making mechanisms slowed and the rats weighed less. The researchers conclude that L-arabinose "inhibits intestinal sucrase activity, thereby reducing sucrose [table sugar] utilization, and consequently decreasing lipogenesis [fat making]."

In other words: L-arabinose can help stop sugar from turning into fat.

CARB-BLOCKER STUDIES
IN DR. PREUSS'S LABORATORY

As an MD, nutritional scientist, and researcher in insulin metabolism, Dr. Preuss was interested in testing the efficacy of carb blockers in his laboratory at Georgetown University Medical Center. He wanted to test three of the ingredients you've just read about: white kidney bean extract, hibiscus extract, and L-arabinose. He also wanted to see what would happen when all three ingredients were combined, in a carb-blocking formula that was already on the market, under the name Carb-Ease.

Here is the hypothesis Dr. Preuss was testing, as formally stated in the published results of the study: "A combination of natural starch blockers and sucrose blockers would diminish and/or slow the absorption of starch and sugar from the intestinal tract, and thus lessen caloric load and ameliorate insulin resistance produced by the rapid absorption of refined carbohydrate."

In other words, carb blockers would actually do all the things we've talked about in this chapter!

So, his next step was to enlist some of his colleagues (and forty-eight rats) and get down to business.

He gave rats one of four different carbohydrates: rice starch, sucrose, glucose, or a combo of rice and sucrose. Then he gave them one of four different carb blockers to respond to those carbohydrate challenges: kidney bean extract, hibiscus extract, L-arabinose, or Carb-Ease. He gave the carb blocker half an hour before and at the time of the challenge. In the hours after the challenge, Dr. Preuss measured glucose levels—as you now know, a good indication of how much carbohydrate has been absorbed.

Remarkable Results

We won't give you every detail of the study—four challenges and four responses make for a lot of neuron-numbing variables that only a statistician could love. But here are the exciting highlights:

Both kidney bean extract and hibiscus were very effective in lowering glucose after the rice starch challenges, as compared to a "control" (a challenge without using a blocker). For example, the average rise in glucose levels two hours after the starch challenge was 46.5 mg/dL in the control rats. But levels only increased by 14.7 with bean and to 5.9 with hibiscus. And higher doses of bean and hibiscus resulted in even lower levels of glucose, when rats were simultaneously challenged with both starch and table sugar.

L-arabinose was very effective in lowering glucose after a sucrose challenge—in fact, there was virtually no glucose in the bloodstream. (As you'd expect for a sugar blocker, it had no measurable effect after a starch challenge.)

Carb-Ease—the combination of white bean extract, hibiscus, and L-arabinose—was dramatically effective. At the highest dosage, there was virtually *no* elevation of circulating glucose levels in the rats challenged with either starch or sucrose.

Long-Term Success

Dr. Preuss also conducted longer tests, in which rats were given infusions of either water or Carb-Ease for nine weeks.

In week 5, sugar was added to the rats' drinking water. The control rats started to develop high blood pressure, while the rats given Carb-Ease had only very slight increases. (Fifty percent of people with insulin resistance have high blood pressure, and studies show the more insulin resistant you are, the higher your blood pressure is likely to be.)

Between weeks 7 and 9, the rats were given the carbohydrate challenges. In rats receiving Carb-Ease, the rise in glucose levels after the starch challenge was approximately half that of controls.

Blood glucose levels after the sucrose challenge were also significantly less in the Carb-Ease rats.

And overall—even when they weren't being specifically challenged with carbohydrate—the Carb-Ease rats had lower levels of blood glucose.

Both the short- and long-term results confirmed the study's hypothesis:

- Carb blockers slow the absorption of refined carbohydrates.

- Carb blockers prevent insulin resistance brought on by the high intake of refined carbohydrates.

Two Not-So-Little Pigs

There was only one problem with this study: the dosages Dr. Preuss was giving to rats were, gram for gram, way too high to give to people. He needed to find out if the typical dosages in an over-the-counter carb blocker would have the same effect as the high doses the rats got. So he conducted the same type of challenge/carb-blocker study on two Yorkshire pigs, weighing 150 and 200 pounds.

He challenged the pigs with sucrose, starch, or a combination of the two, each time giving them a dose of Carb-Ease comparable to the recommended dose for us humans. In each case, Carb-Ease lowered the blood level of glucose after the carb challenge.

(And Dr. Preuss is happy to report that the two male pigs—fondly named Harry and Bobby, the first names of Dr. Preuss and one of the technicians who helped conduct the study—are now living high on the hog at an animal sanctuary in Maryland.)

NATURAL FAT-LOSS PHARMACY
SUCCESS STORY

From 326 to 170 pounds

Michelle M. is a thirty-nine-year-old wife and stay-at-home mom who lives on Hawaii's Big Island. Since her childhood, achieving a healthy weight hasn't been easy for Michelle. She tried to shed the extra pounds, but always felt that she was genetically disposed to gain weight. "For many years, I've watched my mother's weight go up and down, and I saw how my mother's sister struggled with morbid obesity until she died at a young age," Michelle told us. "I knew I had to find something that worked for me, something that would help me win my struggle with weight."

Several years ago she began her search for an effective weight-loss solution, trying popular programs with prepackaged foods, and even the diet drug fen-phen, which has since been recalled. None of these provided the long-term solution she was looking for. "For a while I was successful, but as soon as I stopped eating the prepackaged food, I started gaining weight again. I needed a program that was less rigid, something that I could stick with."

In 1998 she became pregnant with her first child. "I stopped using fen-phen and started gaining weight during my pregnancy. By the end of the pregnancy I had gained 60 pounds! Then, after I had my son, I only lost about 20 pounds of that extra weight. I had been eating way too much, and my weight ballooned."

Another setback came about a year later, when an accident left Michelle with two broken bones in her lower leg. Recovery was long and painful, and the resulting inactivity contributed to additional weight gain. Right around the time her leg began to heal, she became pregnant with her second child. By the end of the pregnancy she had reached her highest weight: 326 pounds.

"I found myself in a very frustrating situation. Here I am, inactive and out of shape, still experiencing pain from the rod that had been placed in my broken leg, trying to take care of two young children. In addition, we had recently moved from San Francisco to Hawaii, so I was in a new place where I had no help from family or friends. I was starting to feel like it was all too much for me to handle."

She read the book *Sugar Busters*, which she had borrowed from a friend, and decided to adopt an eating plan that eliminated most, if not all, of the refined sugars from her diet.

"The first couple of weeks on the Sugar Busters diet were really difficult," she remembers. "I survived, but it showed me how much I craved sugary foods, and starchy foods like potatoes and pasta. I felt as though I was addicted to these foods, almost like I was in withdrawal for a while." After a few weeks, the cravings subsided. "I was sticking to the program and losing weight . . . I got down to around 225 pounds and that was where I hit a plateau."

Once again, health problems began to demand Michelle's attention and her focus shifted away from the stringent eating plan. She was seeing an acupuncturist for recurring back pain and was having continued difficulty with her leg, which was accidentally rebroken when surgeons attempted to remove the rod that had been previously inserted. All this contributed to inactivity and a renewed sense of failure in achieving her weight-loss goals.

Then, in August 2003, she heard about starch blockers. "My acupuncturist knew how frustrated I was, and recommended I try a type of dietary supplement called a 'starch blocker.' I began taking the supplement in pill form before each meal and I started losing weight again.

"The starch blocker helps reduce the amount of calories from starch that are absorbed by the body, so I knew I could still eat starchy foods in moderation. I didn't feel like a failure if I ate some sourdough bread or potatoes, like I did on other diets. Before, if I ate some bread, I'd say to myself, 'Well, I've already screwed up my diet today, I might as well go on and have the pasta and cake as well.' The starch blocker keeps me from this crazy binge cycle, because I know I can eat small amounts of bread, potatoes, or pasta and still lose weight."

Michelle used a starch blocker in conjunction with moderate levels of physical activity, as her leg finally began to heal. "We live on a ten-acre ranch in Hawaii, and I became quite active with the horses, walking them and caring for them a lot during the week. I also found myself drinking more water, since I would drink a glass each time I took a starch blocker, and this certainly improved my health."

Since she's reached her target weight, Michelle now uses her starch blocker on a maintenance basis, taking three or so a week whenever she eats a starchy meal. "I'm down to 170 pounds now, and that's right where I want to be. I never want to go back to looking and feeling overweight and unhealthy."

Carb-Blocking Conclusion

And that leads us to what we think is the only logical conclusion from all the evidence presented in this chapter:

If you want to lose fat and retain muscle, add a carb blocker to your diet and exercise program—it will help you overcome overweight and insulin resistance.

HOW TO USE A CARB BLOCKER

Taking a carb blocker is as easy as . . . well, as the prudent portion of pie you might enjoy eating after you take it.

A few tips to maximize effectiveness:

Take it with an 8-ounce glass of water. This will help your body absorb and use the supplement.

Take it with a meal. Right before or during the meal is best.

Take an effective dose. In Dr. Preuss's research, he found effective per-meal doses are likely to be: 300 milligrams (mg) of bean extract, 600 mg of hibiscus extract, and 500 mg of L-arbinose. But the safest advice is: follow the dosage recommendation on the label of the product you choose to take.

Don't be afraid of long-term use. Is the product safe for long-term use? Obviously, it would be best if there were long-term, large-scale clinical studies on carb blockers. But there aren't. However—given that big doses are safe in animals . . . that there are no side effects in small clinical studies . . . and that there has been a decade of problem-free use in the marketplace—carb blockers seem quite safe. In fact, some—like L-arabinose and hibiscus—are currently used in foods as flavor enhancers.

Keep in mind, carb blockers are not a miracle. There are no nutritional miracles. You can't eat a pint of ice cream and take a carb blocker and expect your weight and blood sugar to be A-okay. Carb blockers are an *aid* to a balanced diet. They give you a little more dietary leeway, so that you don't have to stick to an excessively low-carb diet in order to lose fat and preserve muscle.

CHOOSING A PRODUCT

Deciding to take a carb blocker is the first step. Deciding *which* carb blocker to take is the (potentially bewildering) second. Because once you start checking out the store shelves and the Web sites, you'll quickly find that there are many products to choose from. Which one of them is best for you? The criterion Dr. Preuss uses for choosing a supplement: Pick the ingredients and/or brands used in the studies that proved the supplement's effectiveness. In this case, that includes: Phase 2 (a starch-blocker ingredient found in many products), Carb-Ease, or Carbo-Slim. (Remember: don't take Carbo-Slim if you've got a wheat allergy.)

Some products that contain Phase 2 include:

Best Weight Control Formulas Phase 2 (Swanson)

Carb Blaster (Herbs of Gold)

Carb Counters (Dixie USA)

Carb Cutter (Health and Nutrition Systems International)

Carb Erase (Fitness Labs)

Carb Extractor (HealthSource Inc.)

Carb Intercept and Carb Intercept Chewable (Natrol)

Carbohydrate Blocker (Source Naturals)

CarboTame (Jarrow Formulas)

Carb Phaser 1000 (Biochem)

Carb Shredder (Vitamin Shoppe)

CarbSpa (TrimSpa)

Carb Terminator (NX Generation)

Carb Trim (Quantum)

Maximum Strength Carb Eliminator (Baywood)

Phase 2 (Doctor's A-Z)

Phase 2 (Greenville Health Products)

Phase 2 (Healthy Origins)

Phase 2 (Natural Balance)

Phase 2 (Nature's Harmony)

Phase 2 (Now)

Simple Steps Carb-Down (FoodScience of Vermont)

Starch Blocker (CVS)

Starch Blocker (Good Neighbor Pharmacy)

Starch Control (Nature's Blend)

StarchStopper (Diet World)

Starch Stopper (Innovite)   Walker Diet Carb Block with
TheraSlim (ProThera)   Phase 2 (VitaCost)

So go ahead and try that new risotto dish at the Italian restaurant around the corner. Just don't forget to take your pills!

PART IV

Fat Blockers

Stop Fat from Getting to You

7

- Chitosan and Other Soluble Fibers

Believe it or not, oil spills have had an upside. In their efforts to clean up the mess, scientists concocted *chitosan*, a pulverized powder made from chitin, the outer covering, or exoskeleton, of marine animals like shrimp and crab. This ultra-absorbent powder is spread over the surface of the ocean, where it soaks up oil, grease, and heavy metals, making them easier to remove.

Nutritional scientists were intrigued by chitosan. They figured it might also soak up oils and grease (i.e., fat) in another watery environment: the intestinal tract. And they were basically right. But chitosan doesn't work inside your body like it does when it's floating on oily waves . . .

FAT DIGESTION 101

To understand how chitosan traps fat inside the body, you need to know a little bit about how fat is digested. Basically, there are four steps: (a) In the stomach, acids break down the food you just ate, including fats. (b) In the small intestine, enzymes (proteins that help with chemical reactions) grind fats even finer: into *fatty acids* (the basic components of fat) and tiny fat globules called *monoglycerides*. (c) We're still in the small intestine—and getting ready to digest. On the scene are bile acids, a component of bile, the digestive juice manufactured by the liver and stored in the gallbladder. Bile acids combine with fatty acids and monoglycerides to form *micelles*, fat particles suspended in water so they can be . . . (d) absorbed through the intestinal wall.

Fat digestion has occurred. What happens when you add chitosan to this process? Less fat digestion might occur. Maybe a lot less.

The Fiber Factor

Chitosan, remember, is made from the outer coverings of marine animals. And it's very similar to another outer covering: bran, or cellulose, the indigestible outer covering of grains. In other words, like bran, chitosan is a *fiber*.

A characteristic of all fibers is that they can't be absorbed, or digested. (We'll use the words *absorbed* and *digested* interchangeably throughout this chapter.)

Additionally, chitosan is what's called a *soluble fiber*: it dissolves in water. (*Insoluble* fibers, like wheat bran, don't dissolve.)

In the stomach, soluble chitosan begins dissolving in the acidy soup, breaking up into little pieces. Those chunks of chitosan soak up water, forming globules of sticky gel—which, like nets, surround and capture fats and oils.

In the small intestine, chitosan becomes insoluble: it no longer absorbs water. And it's in the small intestine where another unique chemical property of chitosan goes to work.

Chitosan is *positively charged*, like the positive pole of a magnet. Fatty acids and bile acids are *negatively charged*. Like the negative pole of a magnet to the positive pole of another magnet, they're pulled irresistibly to chitosan. And once the fatty acids and bile acids are attached, they don't detach—and some get a free ride all the way out of the body.

Farewell, fat-creating fatty acids!

Good-bye, fat-digesting bile acids!

And while your body is saying good-bye to all that fat and those fat-making biochemicals, it's also saying good-bye to some *calories*.

Each gram of fat you eat equals 9 calories. (The "average" person eats about 80 to 90 grams of fat a day.) Each gram of chitosan you take can trap a couple of grams of fat. Let's do the fat math: take 3 grams of chitosan a day, and you might avoid digesting 6 to 10 grams of fat, or about 55 to 90 calories. Do that every day for a year, and you'll lose about 9 pounds.

Can any supplement really do that? Scientific studies show chitosan is for real.

STOPPING FAT BEFORE IT STARTS

The first studies on chitosan were conducted using laboratory animals. Scientists were trying to answer two questions:

Did chitosan work? And if so, how?

In most of the studies, lab animals like mice or rats were fed a high-fat diet and divided into two groups, with one getting chitosan and the other not. In almost every such study, the animals getting chitosan excreted a lot more fat than the animals not getting chitosan. And they were excreting more because they were absorbing less. Some studies showed that chitosan could cut fat absorption in half.

Scientists also discovered the mechanism by which chitosan captures fat, as we described earlier: it traps fat in a gel, and binds with negatively charged fatty acids and bile acids.

And there was another positive discovery: animals getting a high-fat diet and chitosan had lower levels of cholesterol than animals not getting chitosan.

The next question scientists wanted to answer: Can chitosan trap fat in people?

The Unappetizing but Inspiring Facts About Chitosan and . . . Fat Excretion

There's no way around it: to present the scientific proof about the effectiveness of chitosan as a fat trapper in people, we have to bring up a topic that's not fit for polite dinner conversation—or for any dinner conversation. Fecal fat excretion. Pardon us while we explain.

To prove whether or not chitosan is "trapping" fat in people, scientists: (1) enlist a bunch of people for a study; (2) divide them into two groups; (3) give one group chitosan and the other a placebo; (4) measure the amount of fat each group eats; and (5) measure the amount of fat each group excretes.

If chitosan is working—if it's trapping fat so it can't be digested—the group taking the supplement will excrete significantly more fat than the group not taking the supplement.

And that's just what many studies on chitosan show.

(Some don't, of course. Scientific proof is never a shutout. That's why there's always more than one point of view about any claim for a pill, product, or approach that is touted to help people lose weight. But when it comes to chitosan, says Dr. Preuss, the majority of the evidence indicates that fat calories are absorbed.)

Absorbed—30 percent fewer fatty acids. In a 1995 study by Japanese researchers, published in *Microbial Ecology in Health and Disease*, people who took chitosan had a 30 percent increase in the excretion of fatty acids after two weeks.

Digested—38 percent less fat. In a 1997 study conducted by Dr. Preuss and his colleagues, people taking chitosan had 38 percent more fat excretion than a placebo group after twelve days of supplementation.

Blocked—34 fat calories a day. Dr. Preuss conducted a second study on chitosan, published in 2002 in the *Journal of Medicine*. Twenty-one people took 2.1 grams of chitosan (along with psyllium, another fiber) during one part of the study, and a placebo during another. While on the chitosan/psyllium combo, they excreted 3.8 more grams of fat a day than while on the placebo. That's 34 fat calories that didn't get a chance to turn into body fat.

Three times more fat snared. In a study published in 2001 in the *Journal of the American Nutraceutical Association*, researchers found average fat excretion increased by 6 grams in a group getting chitosan, compared to a 2-gram decrease in a placebo group.

Fast food, reduced fat. In a 2000 study, researchers gave 1 gram of chitosan each to thirteen people, five to ten minutes before they ate a fatty meal from a fast-food restaurant. After the meal, they measured their levels of triglycerides, a blood fat that is an indicator of fat absorption. Nine out of thirteen had decreases in fat absorption, compared to their standard increase after eating fat. In five people, absorption dropped from 20 to 28 grams. That's 180 to 250 calories!

Now, we're not trying to give you carte blanche to pop a chitosan pill and run out to Wendy MacKing's and order a triple-cheese Mega-Burger. But this study does give you a good idea of chitosan's remarkable power to block fat.

Creamed by chitosan. In a study from Sweden, researchers at Maimo University Hospital gave twelve volunteers 1.7 ounces (50 milliliters) of cream—and then gave them either 1.9 grams of chitosan or a placebo. Over the next five hours, the researchers used a sophisticated method of breath analysis to measure how much fat was being absorbed. The chitosan group absorbed an average of 13 percent less fat than the placebo group, with most chitosan takers absorbing about 25 percent less.

FAT BLOCKED, POUNDS LOST

Okay: it's great that fat was *trapped*. But let's get down to the nitty-fatty. Did anybody lose weight? Yes: pound after pound, year after year. Let's look at the evidence.

The first study. In 1994, Norwegian researchers conducted the first study to see if chitosan could outperform a placebo in helping people lose weight.

Nineteen people on a low-calorie diet took either 1.92 grams of chitosan or a placebo for twenty-eight days. Those on chitosan lost more weight than those on the placebo.

Viva chitosan. Six studies from Italy followed. They were conducted in 1995 and 1996 by thirteen different researchers at five different institutions, and published in *Acta Toxicologica et Therapeutica*. In the studies, anywhere from 30 to 150 people went on a low-calorie diet for twenty-eight days, with half taking chitosan and half a placebo. In *all* of the studies, the chitosan group lost significantly more weight. For example, in one study, those on the placebo lost 4 percent of their weight, while those on chitosan lost 13 percent.

A fiber combo. In 1998, a team of researchers gave 176 people either a placebo or Biozan (a combination of fibers, including chitosan, oat fiber, and beta glucan, a fiberlike substance derived from baker's yeast). Those taking Biozan lost significantly more weight and more body fat than the placebo group.

Almost double the weight loss. In a study conducted in 2000, 322 people who weren't dieting took chitosan. Two-thirds responded very well to the supplement, losing an average of 9 pounds. Overall, the average weight loss was 5 pounds.

A great holiday gift—no weight gain. Chitosan may help you *prevent* weight gain when you need help the most: during the winter holidays. In a study conducted in November and December of 2000, overweight people who weren't dieting took either chitosan or a placebo. The placebo group gained 3.3 pounds. The chitosan group *lost* 2.2 pounds.

Thirty-two percent greater weight loss. In a 2001 study, reported by Polish researchers at the Fourth Conference of the European Chitin Society, fifty overweight women went on a low-calorie diet (1,000 calories a day) for two months, with half taking 4.5 grams of chitosan a day and half taking a placebo. The placebo group lost 24 pounds, while the chitosan group lost 35 pounds—that's 32 percent more weight lost. (Or think of it this way: for every 2 pounds the placebo group lost, the chitosan group lost 3 pounds.)

"Chitosan can be used as a valuable and safe adjuvant in the long-term dietary treatment of obesity," the researchers concluded.

Less Fat on the Body, Less Fat in the Blood

If chitosan traps fat in the stomach and intestines, might it not also lower levels of heart-hurting *blood* fats, like cholesterol and triglycerides? The answer is yes. Let's look at one impressive study, conducted by Italian researchers in 1996.

At the beginning and end of a twenty-eight-day study on chitosan and weight loss, Italian researchers also measured blood fats. Specifically, they looked at total cholesterol; LDL cholesterol (the "bad" cholesterol found in arterial plaque); HDL cholesterol (the "good" cholesterol that carries fat away from the arteries to the liver for disposal); and triglycerides (high levels of this blood fat translate into a higher risk for heart disease).

All the participants in the study ate a very low-calorie (and therefore low-fat) diet, which naturally lowered cholesterol and triglyceride levels. But while blood fats fell in those getting a placebo, they *plummeted* in those getting chitosan. Compared to the placebo group, the chitosan group had a:

- 17 percent greater reduction in total cholesterol

- 20 percent greater reduction in LDL

- 13 percent greater reduction in triglycerides

- 8 percent greater increase in HDL

In a 2002 review of numerous scientific studies looking at the "cholesterol-lowering properties" of chitosan, Finnish scientists point out that the fiber has reduced total cholesterol levels from 6 to 43 percent and levels of LDL cholesterol from 15 to 35 percent.

How does chitosan lower cholesterol?

Chitosan binds with bile acids. Bile acids play a major role in the synthesis of cholesterol. A lower level of bile acids in the body translates into a lower production of total and LDL cholesterol. It also translates into *more* HDL, as the body goes into a bit of overdrive trying to synthesize the "good" variety of cholesterol.

Lower total cholesterol, LDL, and triglycerides, and higher HDL—not a bad "side effect" from a weight-loss supplement.

Chitosan, Xenical, and Alli: They all block fat, but *very* differently

You might think that because chitosan blocks fat, it works much the same way as the fat-blocking prescription drug Xenical (orlistat) and Alli, its new OTC version. Not so.

Xenical and Alli work by attaching to and partially disabling *lipase*, an enzyme that breaks down fat for digestion. About 30 percent less fat is digested, and the undigested fat is excreted.

Chitosan works in a completely different way, as described earlier. In the stomach, chitosan forms a gel, entrapping fat particles. In the intestine, positively charged chitosan attracts negatively charged fatty acids and bile acids (like the positive pole of a magnet attracts the negative pole of another magnet): the fatty acids and bile acids are bound to the indigestible chitosan and never get absorbed.

And there's another way Xenical, Alli, and chitosan differ. Chitosan has never been shown to have significant side effects. Xenical has.

Xenical has common, bothersome GI-adverse reactions, according to Sidney Wolfe, MD, the director of Public Citizen's Health Research Group. They include, he says, "oily spotting, gas with discharge, fecal urgency, fatty/oily stools, and frequent bowel movements." And, he points out, Xenical also reduces the absorption of so-called fat-soluble vitamins, like A, D, E, and K.

Those are problems you're much less likely to have with chitosan.

CHITOSAN: PRO AND CON

As we said earlier, not every scientist is a fan of chitosan. Researchers from the Department of Nutrition at the University of California at Davis, for example, studied chitosan and fat absorption. Writing in the *Journal of the American Dietetic Association*, they conclude: "This product . . . fails to meet claims." What's going on? Is chitosan really cheatosan?

There are a couple of reasons why scientists might get negative findings when studying chitosan, says Dr. Preuss. The chitosan used may not be of the highest quality. The dosages may be too low. The people studied might not have taken chitosan at the best time, right before meals. But, says Dr. Preuss, for all the naysaying, many of the studies on chitosan and weight loss have produced positive results. "While some could quibble with each individual study," he says, "the overall impression is that chitosan works."

THE BEST WAY TO TAKE CHITOSAN

How can you make sure chitosan works for you?

Take the right dose. Scientific studies have used from 1 to 10 grams a day. For example, the Italian researchers who studied people on a 1,000-calorie-a-day diet used about 1 gram of chitosan. But if you eat more calories, you're probably going to need more chitosan. Dr. Preuss recommends 3 grams a day as a prudent dose.

At the right time. Chitosan works by hobbling the fat you just ate. That's why you should take it five to thirty minutes before a meal. Take 1 gram before each meal.

With plenty of water. In the stomach, chitosan absorbs water, forming a gel. So make sure there's some water in there: take a chitosan supplement with an 8-ounce glass of water. And no sipping—make sure you drink the whole thing! If you don't, you could suffer dehydration of the GI tract, or even an impaction.

Pick a reliable product. There are many, many (did we say *many*?) brands of chitosan supplements on the shelves. Some products, however, might have a slight edge: they're *deacetylated*, allowing them to dissolve more quickly in stomach acid and possibly absorb more fat. And, says Dr. Preuss, a type of chitosan called LipoSan Ultra may be the deacetylated variety that's most effective. Brands with LipoSan Ultra include: Now, Natural Balance, Nutraceutical Sciences Institute, and Swanson.

SAFE AS SEAFOOD

Is a substance widely used in the pharmaceutical, food, agricultural, and cosmetics industries likely to be unsafe? No.

Is a substance given to thousands of people in dozens of clinical trials, without any significant side effects, likely to be unsafe? No.

Is a substance that has been on the market for a decade or more, and has been taken by over a million people—again, without any significant side effects—likely to be unsafe? No.

Of course, *any* substance can be dangerous in very high doses, even water. But when toxicology studies on chitosan (to see if it was *toxic*, or poisonous) were conducted in mice, chitosan did not become deadly until the animals received a daily dose of 16 grams per kilogram (2.2 pounds) of body weight. That would be like a person weighing 150 pounds taking over 1,000 grams a day, or three hundred times the recommended dose.

Chitosan does have one safety issue: it's made from the shells of shrimp and crab. So if you're allergic to seafood you may be allergic to chitosan. Case in point: in one study on chitosan, 2 to 3 percent of the people taking it had an allergic reaction—and almost all of them were allergic to seafood. If you're allergic to seafood, stay away from chitosan.

CHITOSAN OF ALL TRADES

Chitosan is a *very* versatile fiber, used in many different ways.

Pharmaceuticals. Chitosan is used widely in the pharmaceutical industry, both *as* a medicine and as an ingredient *in* medicines to help them work better. As a topical medicine, chitosan can help skin regenerate, healing burns and wounds. It is used in artificial skin, corneal dressing, surgical sutures, and dental implants. It's been shown to reduce dental bacteria, and to help stop vaginal infections like *Candida albicans* and chlamydia.

As an ingredient, it masks bitter tastes in medicines. It also helps with drug delivery and time release, making sure a medicine gets to the right part of the body at the right time.

Food industry. Chitosan is used as a thickener and stabilizer to help sauces keep their consistency. It's a *flocculating agent*, helping beverages stay clear rather than turn cloudy. It's also used as a preservative.

Agriculture. Chitosan is used as a coating for seeds, to protect them against frost. It's combined with fertilizers and nutrients for time release into soil. And because it's antimicrobial, it's sprayed on fruits and vegetables to keep them free of bacteria and fungus.

Cosmetics. Chitosan forms a protective, moisturizing, flexible film on skin, and also combines with other ingredients to help them do the same. For that reason, it's widely used in moisturizers and sunscreens. It's also used in shampoos and hairsprays, mainly for its antibacterial effect.

FIBER: THE BIG PICTURE

Chitosan—derived from the exoskeleton of sea animals, and positively charged—is an unusual fiber. But even typical fibers—the indigestible portion of a plant, whether it's the bran of a wheat kernel, the husk of a seed, or the skin of a fruit—may also help you lose weight. Fiber can:

- Help you feel satisfied sooner when you eat, so you eat less. (In fact, no fewer than seventeen scientific studies have shown that fiber improves *satiety*, the feeling that your appetite has been satisfied and you're ready to stop eating.)

- Stop some of the calories you just ate from being absorbed.

- Help you feel less hungry in the hours after a meal.

But if you're like the typical American, you're not getting too many of those benefits from high-fiber *foods*.

The government recommends men get 38 grams a day of fiber and women 25. But the average intake for men is only 17 grams, and for women only 13. (It's not that men are more fiber-conscious. They just eat more.) Many *dieters* are even more fiber-deprived. According to a study in the *Journal of the American College of Nutrition*, the Atkins diet provides about 4 grams of fiber a day.

The Lower the Fiber Intake, the Higher the Weight

If you're getting an F minus on your fiber report card, you may be seeing higher numbers on the scale. Join the club.

Swedish researchers studied 5,000 people and found those who were overweight ate the fewest fiber-rich foods.

Canadian doctors found that people who weren't overweight ate an average of 19 grams of fiber a day, while overweight people typically ate 14.

Researchers in Indiana discovered a similar trend: normal-weight men ate an average of 27 grams of fiber a day and normal-weight women 23, while overweight men ate 21 grams and overweight women 16.

Researchers in England matched fiber intake and body mass index (BMI, a measure of body fat) in more than 5,000 people: the lower the fiber intake, the higher the BMI.

Boston researchers, reporting their results in the *Journal of the American Medical Association*, found a similar correlation among nearly 3,000 young men: the lower the fiber intake, the higher the weight. The researchers also analyzed weight *regain* over ten years among the men who had lost weight. Those who ate the most fiber gained back the least weight.

Norwegian researchers gave either a 6-gram fiber supplement or a placebo to fifty-three overweight women who were on a 1,200-calorie diet for six months. The fiber group lost 18 pounds, while the placebo group lost 13.

Researchers at Tufts University in Boston reviewed *all* the published studies on fiber and weight loss. In their report in *Nutrition Reviews*, they say the majority of studies prove that fiber increases the feeling of satisfaction that leads you to stop eating (satiety) and decreases hunger in the hours after a meal. The studies also show that, if you're overweight, adding 14 grams per day of fiber to your diet helps you eat about 18 percent fewer calories and lose an extra 5 pounds over four months. And, they point out, you get this positive result whether you add the fiber from foods or a fiber supplement. Increasing dietary fiber, they conclude, "may help decrease the currently high national prevalence of obesity."

Should you take a fiber supplement?

Food First, Supplement Second

To help answer that question, we talked to Joanne L. Slavin, PhD, RD, a professor in the Department of Food Science and Nutrition at the University of Minnesota, and an expert in fiber and weight loss.

Dr. Slavin recommends that you first try to increase your intake of *dietary fiber*, by eating more whole grains, vegetables, fruits, and beans. But if those foods aren't a major portion of your menu—and for most people they're not, and they're not going to be—she recommends taking the next step. "I would suggest a fiber supplement for people who are not meeting the recommended intake of fiber," she told us.

What kind of supplement?

Her top recommendation (and also that of Dr. Preuss) is to take a supplement with a *mix* of fibers, which could include chitosan. But she says that any fiber supplement that is "convenient and works with the person's food intake" (in other words, a supplement you actually take every day, day after day) is the right supplement.

She recommends taking the supplement three times a day, with meals.

And, of course, she emphasizes that you need to drink plenty of water each time you take the supplement, just as you should with chitosan.

And—as with *all* the supplements recommended in *The Natural Fat-Loss Pharmacy*—she says fiber supplements only work as *part* of a weight-loss plan that includes a healthy diet and regular exercise.

A Fiber Supplement That's All Mixed Up

The type of supplement that Dr. Preuss and Dr. Slavin recommend as their top choice—a mixed fiber supplement—was studied by Dr. Michael Gonzalez and his colleagues at the University of Puerto Rico. The supplement (Fattache) includes chitosan, psyllium, pectin, and gums. (We'll talk more about each one of those fibers in a moment.) Over six weeks, twenty-seven overweight people took either Fattache or a placebo. The fiber group lost an average of 9 pounds; the placebo group, 2.

When Dr. Gonzalez gave the same supplement to overweight kids for six weeks, their average weight dropped from 122 pounds to 116.

"A combination fiber supplement is a safe and effective way to assist in weight reduction," he told us.

Let's look at a few of the fibers besides chitosan that you'll typically find in a weight-loss supplement, either mixed or alone.

Glucomannan

This soluble fiber is derived from the root of elephant yam, or konjac, a plant found in Asia.

More weight loss. Researchers in Norway at the University of Tromso studied 176 healthy, overweight men and women on a 1,200-calorie diet. Some took products containing glucomannan and some a placebo.

Glucomannan-containing supplements "induced significantly more weight reduction than placebo," wrote the researchers, in *Medical Science Monitor*.

Less hunger between meals. In a study conducted by researchers at the University of Rome, thirty overweight people took glucomannan supplements for two months while on a low-calorie diet. When eating, they felt fuller sooner. They were less hungry between meals. They lost weight. And they had decreased cholesterol and blood sugar levels. In fact, many studies show glucomannan can lower cholesterol and balance blood sugar.

Psyllium

This fiber is derived from the seed husks of *P. psyllium*, a variety of plantain. Like chitosan (and all the other fibers discussed in this chapter), it's *soluble*: it forms a soft gel when combined with water. Because that gel adds bulk to stool, it can help clear up a case of constipation, which is why psyllium is the active ingredient in the laxative Metamucil.

Fiber for the first course. French researchers gave psyllium supplements to fourteen people before meals. "Psyllium reduces hunger feelings and energy intake [the amount of food you eat at the meal]," conclude the researchers, in the *European Journal of Clinical Nutrition*.

Balanced blood sugar. In a Spanish study, researchers gave psyllium supplements to overweight children and adolescents. The supplement reduced their cholesterol and balanced their blood sugar. *Hundreds* of other studies report positive results in using psyllium for controlling cholesterol and blood sugar.

Pectin

Pectin is the soluble fiber found in fruit: in the skin of an apple or plum, or the peel of an orange.

SUPPLEMENT SUPPORTER

MARY SHOMON
www.thyroid-info.com

Author, *The Thyroid Diet* and *Living Well with Hypothyroidism*; leading advocate for people with thyroid problems and publisher of the newsletter *Sticking Out Our Necks*

"If you are trying to lose weight and you have hypothyroidism and it is not properly diagnosed and managed—you will not lose weight," says Mary Shomon, author of the *New York Times* bestseller *The Thyroid Diet*, and creator of the Internet's most popular Web site on thyroid problems.

Why not?

Hypothyroidism slows down the metabolism, so you burn fewer calories. It causes fatigue, so you're less apt to exercise. And it triggers the release of stress hormones, which makes you more prone to belly fat.

That's why, she says, every person trying to lose weight should get a diagnosis for thyroid function (on her site you can find a state-by-state list of top thyroid doctors). And, if it turns out you have hypothyroidism, she advises you to follow the weight-loss advice in her book—which includes giving your metabolism a helping hand with weight-loss supplements.

And which weight-loss supplements do people with thyroid problems like to use the most?

CLA, fiber, and hoodia.

"I conducted a poll in *Sticking Out Our Necks*, and 23 percent of readers chose CLA as their favorite weight-loss supplement," she says. Second place went to fiber supplements, at 22 percent, and third place to hoodia, at 17 percent.

Right now, Mary says she's using three weight-loss supplements herself: a fiber supplement, hoodia, and caralluma, an appetite suppressant similar to hoodia. (For more information on hoodia and caralluma, please see Chapter 9, Trying to Solve the Prickly Problem of Appetite.)

"The fiber supplement provides 17 grams of soluble fiber and insoluble fiber," she told us. "I take it before I eat, and it helps fill me up before the meal. I've found this supplement very helpful in losing and maintaining weight."

When we talked to her, she had been taking caralluma for several weeks, and really liking it. "I'm finding that it adds some extra energy and lowers appetite somewhat," she says. "I take it in conjunction with hoodia, and I think the combination really seems to pack an extra punch as far as suppressing appetite."

More satisfied. In a study reported in the *Journal of the American College of Nutrition*, army doctors gave seventy-four soldiers pectin and measured how satisfied they felt when they ate, and how much they ate. The result: "Pectin in doses as small as 5 grams . . . increases satiety and can aid in a program to reduce weight by limiting food intake."

Food sticks around. In a study conducted by researchers in the Department of Medicine at the University of Southern California Medical Center, and reported in *Gastroenterology*, pectin helped overweight people feel fuller. "Pectin induces satiety [satisfaction] and delays gastric emptying [increasing the amount of time food stays in the stomach] in obese patients, and may be a useful adjuvant [addition] in the treatment of disorders of overeating."

Guar Gum

This soluble fiber is derived from the seeds of the guar plant (*Cyamopsis tetragonolobus*), which grows in India and Pakistan. It's been successfully used to treat constipation, diarrhea, and irritable bowel syndrome.

Feeling fuller. In a study by Dutch researchers, published in the *European Journal of Clinical Nutrition*, taking guar gum before a meal helped overweight people feel fuller.

However, in an article published in the *American Journal of Medicine*, scientists from the University of Exeter in Britain reviewed twenty studies of guar gum and weight loss and concluded the fiber was *not* a good option, not only because it didn't work, but also because it has side effects like stomach pain, gas, diarrhea, and cramps.

The Fiber Finish

"Supplemental fibers show promise as aids to weight loss," says Dr. Slavin. "Moreover," she says, "consumers who choose low-carbohydrate, high-protein diets to aid in weight loss should consider supplemental dietary fiber to help close the fiber gap."

Ditto from Dr. Preuss. Whether you choose chitosan, a mixed fiber supplement, or another soluble fiber—a bit of bulk can be one of a dieter's best friends.

PART V

Appetite Suppressors

Natural Control for Food Cravings

8

- ## 5-HTP (5-Hydroxy-L-Tryptophan)

You've no doubt heard of (or perhaps taken) Prozac, Sarafem, Paxil, Zoloft, Celexa, Luvox, or one of the other *selective serotonin reuptake inhibitors* (SSRIs) commonly prescribed for depression or anxiety. Serotonin is a *neurotransmitter*, a chemical that helps neurons—the cells of the brain—transmit messages to one another. An SSRI reduces the amount of serotonin reabsorbed by brain cells, leaving more around for cell-to-cell transmission. And that's literally a good idea.

When your brain has enough serotonin, your mood is likely to be good—you feel less anxious and depressed. You're calmer and more relaxed, so you have a better chance of getting a good night's sleep. While pain is never good, it may not be as bad when serotonin levels are high enough. (For example, serotonin can mute migraines.) But serotonin not only affects mood—it also affects *food*.

With sufficient serotonin, your appetite is likely to be balanced: when you eat, you feel satisfied sooner. And you're less likely to crave (and binge on) carbohydrates. Or raid the refrigerator when you feel stressed. And that's saying a lot. Because it's these very problems—never feeling really full; overdoing it on sugary, starchy foods; eating to relieve stress—that can sabotage the well-meaning but often failed efforts of millions of people to lose weight.

How can you get more serotonin into your brain—and keep it there?

SSRIs are, of course, one common solution: doctors write approximately 150 million prescriptions for SSRIs every year, some of them to help with eating disorders or overweight. In fact, the infamous prescription medication Redux, or fen-phen—banned for damaging heart valves—worked by boosting serotonin levels.

Meridia (sibutramine)—the most commonly prescribed weight-loss medication on the market—also works by boosting serotonin (and noradrenaline, another neurostransmitter). Like Redux, however, Meridia is not without controversy. In 2002, the consumer group Public Citizen petitioned the FDA to ban the drug, arguing that its effectiveness had never been proven, and pointing out that it had caused 124 hospitalizations for heart problems—along with forty-nine deaths.

An experimental drug, APD356, currently in clinical trials, also works by increasing serotonin. In one study, electrocardiograms showed that there were no heart irregularities among those taking APD356 for one month. But time will tell—and, with prescription drugs, it often tells unpleasant truths about side effects.

(Accomplia, the newest prescription anti-obesity drug to hit the market, also works on brain cells. But it doesn't affect serotonin. It blocks *cannabinoid receptors*, the part of the cell responsible for the carb-mad "munchies" experienced by some users of cannabis, or marijuana.)

As you can see, serotonin-boosting prescription drugs seem like a slightly unsafe bet for weight loss. Is there a *safe* way to increase your levels of serotonin and control carb cravings and overeating?

Yes. The amino acid, 5-HTP.

WHY NOT TAKE L-TRYPTOPHAN?

Serotonin's chemical cognomen is a tongue twister: 5-hydroxyl-tryptamine, or 5-HT, for short. It's formed as the final step in a complex biochemical process that starts with the essential amino acid L-tryptophan, found in foods like meat, cottage cheese, peanuts, and sesame seeds. L-tryptophan is then converted to another amino acid: 5-hydroxy-L-tryptophan: 5-HTP. And 5-HTP then becomes serotonin. In brief: L-tryptophan to 5-HTP to serotonin.

If L-tryptophan is the first step in the creation of serotonin, why not take an L-tryptophan supplement? Why take 5-HTP? To answer that question, let's travel back in time to October 1989.

The Strange Case of EMS

Three doctors in New Mexico each saw a different patient afflicted with a mysterious illness. All three of the patients had severe "myalgia" (muscle and joint pain), along with some combination of various other symptoms, like cough, chills, weakness, mouth ulcers, and skin rash. Blood work revealed that each person also had a very high level of a certain type of white blood cell (called an eosinophil). The doctors reported these cases to the New Mexico Health and Environmental Department, and the department reported them to the federal government's Centers for Disease Control and Prevention—which soon began getting reports from all over the country about this strange and sometimes deadly condition.

Eventually, over 1,500 cases were reported, including forty-six deaths. The condition was dubbed the eosinophilia-myalgia syndrome, or EMS. And medical detective work revealed that all individuals with EMS had something in common: they were all taking L-tryptophan.

In November 1989, the Food and Drug Administration recalled all the L-tryptophan on the market. However, later research revealed that the amino acid *wasn't* to blame. In every case of EMS, the patient had been taking L-tryptophan manufactured at a particular facility in Japan. It turned out that their product was *contaminated*: a new strain of bacteria used in the fermentation process that creates L-tryptophan supplements had been inadvertently allowed to run rampant because of several shortcuts in the company's purification and filtering processes. But this dark cloud of disease and death had a silver lining.

"One very positive development arising from the EMS crisis was that it led to a search for a nonprescription alternative to L-tryptophan," says Michael Murray, ND, a naturopathic physician, faculty member of Bastyr University in Seattle, Washington, and author of twenty books, including *5-HTP: The Natural Way to Overcome Depression, Obesity, and Insomnia.*

As you've probably guessed by now, that nonprescription alternative was 5-HTP. And it turns out that the body has a *much* easier time converting 5-HTP to serotonin than it does L-tryptophan.

Trying (and Failing) to Turn L-tryptophan into Serotonin

A number of factors can block the conversion of L-tryptophan to serotonin—and it's likely you're experiencing one or more of them. There's . . .

Low levels of vitamin B$_6$. A risk for people over fifty.

Insulin resistance. In this common condition (discussed extensively in the chapters on chromium and on starch and sugar blockers), cells can't make ready use of the hormone insulin, and blood sugar stays high.

Stress. Not much of a problem for you or anybody you know, right?

Low levels of magnesium. The government's recommended "daily value" for magnesium is 400 milligrams (mg) a day, but a survey conducted by the Centers for Disease Control and Prevention found that the average intake was only 290 mg. "Magnesium intake from dietary sources in the U.S. population remains suboptimal," the researchers concluded, in the *Journal of Nutrition.*

It's these and other causes (like lack of exercise, and drinking too much coffee or alcohol) that have created an epidemic of *serotonin deficiency syndrome* in America and around the world, says Dr. Murray. And one "symptom" of that syndrome is overeating carbohydrates and getting fat!

But it's not only lifestyle factors that make 5-HTP the better choice. Biochemistry plays a role, too. Seventy percent of 5-HTP is converted to serotonin, as compared to 3 percent for L-tryptophan. 5-HTP is ushered straight into the brain, while L-tryptophan has to "compete" with other amino acids. And 5-HTP does double duty, raising the levels of various feel-good neurotransmitters, while L-tryptophan affects only serotonin.

And the final convincing fact that 5-HTP is superior to L-tryptophan: numerous studies have shown that 5-HTP actually *works* to calm carbohydrate cravings and help people lose weight. Let's take a look at them.

HOW TO CUT 1,000 CALORIES A DAY—
WITHOUT EVEN TRYING

"5-HTP solves one of the biggest problems that contribute to overweight: serotonin deficiency," Dr. Murray told us. He explains that serotonin signals the brain when the body has eaten enough, a feeling of satisfaction scientists call *satiety*. In short, 5-HTP makes you feel fuller, sooner. It also helps improve your mood, he says, making it easier to stick with a diet and exercise program. And those aren't just claims—those are assertions backed up by scientific proof.

When in Rome, Eat as the Romans Eat

The research on 5-HTP, appetite, and weight loss was conducted by Dr. Filippo Rossi-Fanelli and his team of researchers in the Laboratory of Clinical Nutrition at the University of Rome, in Italy. We talked with Dr. Rossi-Fanelli, who was eager to share with us his insights gleaned from more than a decade of remarkable research into 5-HTP.

STRESS, OVEREATING, AND 5-HTP

What happens to rats when you deprive them of food and then allow them to eat? They eat.

What happens to rats when you stress them out by pinching their tails? They eat.

What happens to those same rats when you give them 5-HTP?

That's what scientists in the Department of Pharmaceutical Sciences at the Massachusetts College of Pharmacy and Health Sciences in Boston were trying to find out. For anybody who overeats when under stress, their results are very encouraging.

The food-deprived rats didn't eat quite as much when they were given 5-HTP—and the more 5-HTP they got, the less food they ate.

But the stressed rats getting 5-HTP also ate less—*eight times less* than the food-deprived rats getting 5-HTP!

In other words, for rats (and maybe for us humans in the daily rat race) 5-HTP is uniquely and powerfully effective in controlling the impulse to eat when stressed.

"5-HTP may be useful in controlling the excessive food intake sometimes generated by stress," wrote the researchers, in the January 2004 issue of *Pharmacology, Biochemistry and Behavior*.

Dr. Rossi-Fanelli began to be interested in 5-HTP after studies on laboratory animals and people in the 1970s and 1980s showed that boosting serotonin levels with L-tryptophan decreased appetite (in animals) and carbohydrate craving (in people). Other studies conducted by Dr. Rossi-Fanelli and his colleagues correlated higher blood levels of L-tryptophan with lack of appetite in cancer patients.

And, he notes, a 1989 study in the prestigious journal *Lancet* showed that serotonin-increasing Redux could help people lose weight—but, he notes ruefully, "with a high incidence of side effects." Ditto, he says, for a study reported in the *American Journal of Psychiatry* in 1990, where forty-five overweight people were given either the SSRI Prozac or a placebo for one year. Those who got the Prozac lost significantly more weight than those who didn't. But they also had significantly more side effects. Could 5-HTP perform as well as Redux or Prozac—*without* the side effects?

Carbs, Calories, and 5-HTP

Dr. Rossi-Fanelli's first study was conducted in 1989. He looked at nineteen very overweight women, with BMIs (body mass index, a measure of overweight) of 30 to 40.

A five-foot-five-inch woman weighing 180 pounds has a BMI of 30. The same woman weighing 240 pounds has a BMI of 40. If that woman had a BMI of 24—a BMI just under what's considered overweight—she would weigh 145 pounds. In other words, the women Dr. Rossi-Fanelli was studying didn't just have a few pounds to lose—they were 35 to 100 pounds overweight.

The women received 8 mg of 5-HTP per kilogram (2.2 pounds) of body weight—the level of intake that Dr. Rossi-Fanelli thinks is best for weight loss. On average, the women took about 600 mg of 5-HTP a day— 200 mg before each meal.

During part of the study, they took 5-HTP, and during another part of the study they took a placebo.

Before the women started taking 5-HTP, the researchers analyzed their food intake, and concluded their main dietary dilemma was not just overeating, but overeating *carbohydrates*.

The researchers didn't restrict what the women were eating—they wanted to see if 5-HTP would have an effect on the amount of calories and carbohydrates they consumed. And it definitely did.

Eating 1,084 Fewer Calories a Day—But Who's Counting?

Before the study started, the women were eating an average of 2,903 calories per day. While on the placebo, they ate 2,327 calories—a definite demonstration of the "placebo effect," or the power of belief to change behavior and health. But while on 5-HTP, the women *really* cut their calories—down to an average of 1,819 per day.

How do those calorie-cutting numbers translate into real-world weight loss? If you ate 1,084 fewer calories a day, you could lose approximately 70 pounds in a year!

Along with their calorie intake, their protein intake dropped: from 101 grams to 79 grams. But their carbohydrate intake *plummeted*: from 274 grams a day to 176.

That's like cutting twenty-five teaspoons of sugar out of your diet every day—without even trying! Some other 100-grams-of-carb comparisons, to give you an idea of how much the women *weren't* eating: 2½ cups of pasta, 4 cups of sugary cereal, 5 crumpets, 4 doughnuts, 6½ slices of white bread, 2½ cups of ice cream, or 30 or 40 large jelly beans. Imagine eliminating that amount of carbs from your daily diet—and not thinking twice about it.

During the study, the women filled out forms rating their level of appetite. They didn't feel any less hungry *before* a meal. But *when* they ate, they felt satisfied sooner—their satiety mechanism was in fifth gear.

Impressed with their results, which were published in the *Journal of Neural Transmission* in 1989, Dr. Rossi-Fanelli and his team decided to see if they could "replicate" them in a second study—a standard scientific process, whereby a new finding is either verified or called into question by additional research.

Again, the researchers looked at overweight overeaters—carb cravers with a BMI of 30 to 40. Again, 5-HTP outperformed the placebo.

In twelve weeks, the women on 5-HTP lost 10.3 pounds; the women on the placebo lost 2.2. The study appeared in the journal *Advances in Experimental Medicine and Biology*, in 1991.

The researchers then conducted a third study, reporting their results in 1992, in the *American Journal of Clinical Nutrition*. And those results were even better than the findings of the first two studies.

Twelve Weeks, Twelve Pounds

Again, Dr. Rossi-Fanelli and his colleagues studied overweight women with BMIs between 30 and 40. Needless to say, every one of those women was eating more calories per day than her body needed to maintain weight.

Again, the women got either 5-HTP or a placebo. They took the supplements right before each meal, with a total intake of 900 mg of 5-HTP per day.

The study lasted twelve weeks. During the first six weeks, the women were allowed to eat whatever they wanted. During the second six weeks, they ate a 1,200-calorie-per-day diet—53 percent carbs, 29 percent fats, and 18 percent protein.

They were weighed every two weeks. And at each two-week interval, they filled out a diet diary (what they ate over the last three days). They also answered a questionnaire about their eating behavior: Were they hungry before meals, or not? Quickly satisfied when they ate, or not? How did different types of food seem to them—appealing, repulsive, or otherwise?

The doctors measured blood chemistry every two weeks, to see if 5-HTP was causing any abnormal changes. And they measured urine levels of 5-HTP, to see if the women were actually taking the supplement.

The results were serotonincredible.

From 219 to 207 pounds. Those taking the placebo hardly lost any weight. They went from an average weight of 207.5 pounds to an average weight of 205.6 pounds—1.9 pounds. Yawn.

In the first six weeks, the 5-HTP group went from an average weight of 219.3 pounds to 215 pounds. By the end of the study, they had gone down to 207.7 pounds, losing almost 12 pounds, or 1 pound per week.

Slashing 1,341 calories a day—and half the carbs. The placebo group didn't cut calories during the first six weeks of unlimited eating *or* the second six weeks—when they were supposed to be on a diet!

But during the first six weeks, when they could eat whatever they wanted to, the 5-HTP group reduced calories by an average of 1,341 per day—including cutting their intake of carbs in half!

Staying power. And during the period when they were supposed to eat a 1,200-calorie diet, the 5-HTP group actually *ate* a 1,200-calorie diet— with an intake of carbohydrates *lower* than what the scientists were recommending.

Remember: these were women who had had just the opposite style of eating for years.

During the first six weeks, all of the women said they felt more satisfied when eating while on 5-HTP; eighteen of the twenty women had that experience during the second six weeks, on the low-calorie diet.

There were no abnormal changes in blood chemistry or any obvious side effects.

The women taking 5-HTP did experience some nausea during the first six weeks of the study, which went away during the second six weeks. (Dr. Murray gave us product recommendations that should eliminate this side effect; we'll discuss them at the end of the chapter.)

The Serotonin Connection

Serotonin, concluded Dr. Rossi-Fanelli and his colleagues, *definitely* plays a major role in eating and satiety. It probably does so by activating brain cells responsible for feeling satisfied when you eat—what he calls the *satiety neurons*.

And it also plays a role in *macronutrient* selection—how much carbohydrate, fat, and protein you decide to eat. And it does that most powerfully in overweight people who eat a lot of carbohydrates.

The women in this study had spent a lifetime overeating carbs. But during the twelve weeks of the study, they spontaneously chose to eat fewer carbohydrates—less pasta and less bread, in particular. (We're talking about Italians, remember.)

In summary, the women taking the 5-HTP:

- Felt fuller, sooner, at every meal.

- Ate fewer carbs, without trying.

- Easily stayed on a low-calorie diet.

- Lost an average of 1 pound a week, for twelve weeks.

Not a bad day's, week's, and month's work for a weight-loss supplement.

"I would recommend 5-HTP to any overweight person who needs to lose weight and who has trouble sticking with a low-calorie diet," Dr. Rossi-Fanelli told us.

DOUBLE DUTY FOR DIABETICS

Dr. Rossi-Fanelli also recommends 5-HTP for non-insulin-dependent, type 2 diabetics—people with the disease who take oral medications but don't have to inject insulin to keep their blood sugar under control. (We're talking about millions of Americans.)

"Taking 5-HTP may help these individuals reduce their carbohydrate intake and thereby improve blood sugar control," he told us. "This may, in turn, delay the progress of their disease, from needing oral antidiabetic medications to needing insulin."

Dr. Rossi-Fanelli isn't making this recommendation out of the blue. In 1998, he and his colleagues published a study in the *International Journal of Obesity*, looking at twenty people with non-insulin-dependent diabetes mellitus (NIDDM). As Dr. Rossi-Fanelli points out, these folks typically overeat and are overweight—and helping them *not* overeat is one of the mainstays of diabetic therapy. And diabetics typically don't overeat anything and everything. *Carbohydrate craving* is the modus operandi(et) of most NIDDM, he says. Getting them to break this habit is usually very slow going, if there's any going at all. Why?

Well, says Dr. Rossi-Fanelli, research shows that people with NIDDM have higher blood levels of amino acids that compete with L-tryptophan

NATURAL FAT-LOSS PHARMACY SUCCESS STORY

Overcoming Out-of-Control Carbohydrate Cravings

Dr. Michael Murray told us this story about one of his patients, a teenage girl who took 5-HTP to overcome the bingeing and purging of bulimia—an eating disorder that many experts think may be caused or complicated by low serotonin levels.

"Jessica was a seventeen-year-old girl with severe bulimia. It was just heartbreaking to see this absolutely beautiful child in such a state—her face was sallow, she had dark rings around her eyes, and her 'smile' was a fixed, flat line.

"When Jessica told me about her problem, I realized that she was a girl in tremendous turmoil. She experienced severe carbohydrate cravings almost every other day. To satisfy them, her item of choice for her binges was heavily sugared breakfast cereal—she would eat two or three large boxes, and then purge. 'I just go into the bathroom, stick my finger down my throat, and throw it all up again,' she said, in an unexpressive voice.

"Her parents brought her to see me after conventional medicine and therapy had failed. I explained my perspective on bulimia to Jessica. I told her that it's a serious, difficult-to-treat illness. Then I described the serotonin system in simple terms.

"I showed her how the emotional stresses she was experiencing—low grades; stopping most of her extracurricular activities, like cheerleading and be-

for entry into the brain, where it turns into serotonin. He theorizes, therefore, that serotonin is lower in NIDDM—and might cause the overeating and carb craving. Could 5-HTP reverse this situation? He decided to find out.

He studied twenty overweight diabetic patients—men and women, aged thirty-five to seventy. For two weeks, one group got 5-HTP: 250 mg, three times a day with meals. The other group got a placebo.

They kept food diaries every day. They also weighed food before meals, reweighing any that was left over. (A "next of kin" had to witness both activities—and sign off!)

ing on the student council; breaking up with her boyfriend—were affecting the chemical balance of her brain, decreasing her levels of serotonin and causing her to feel depressed. I also explained how serotonin affects the appetite control center of the brain, especially those 'switches' that tell her body when it's time to stop eating.

"I prescribed 100 mg of 5-HTP, to be taken three times a day, twenty minutes before meals. I explained my hope that 5-HTP would raise her serotonin levels and curb her cravings. Her response to 5-HTP was amazing. Given the dire nature of her condition, I asked her to call me on Saturday, after she had only been on 5-HTP for four days. She told me that she had never felt better—more in control, with fewer and less intense food cravings, and that she was sleeping better.

"Careful follow-up over the next few months clearly showed that she was no longer bulimic. I ran into her four years later at a coffee shop in Seattle, and it was wonderful to see how well her life was turning out—she was a healthy and happy young adult!"

"The brain chemistry pattern in bulimia and binge-eating disorders is quite interesting," Dr. Murray told us. "When they binge, these people literally get an unbelievable rush of feel-good chemicals in their brains, including serotonin. But this effect is short-lived. By improving brain chemistry through its conversion to serotonin, 5-HTP is often able to reduce the factors that trigger the need for binge eating—as well as provide a less dramatic but more sustainable feeling of pleasure *without* bingeing."

The researchers also took blood measurements that would indicate whether the diabetics had lower-than-normal levels of L-tryptophan available to the brain for conversion to serotonin.

Fewer Calories a Day

Calorie reduction. The placebo group didn't eat any fewer calories during the two weeks of the study. But after the first week, the 5-HTP group had cut their average daily intake from 1,926 calories to 1,521. By the end of the second week, it was down to 1,507.

Carb reduction, too. The placebo group didn't have any change in the consumption of *macronutrient*—they were eating the same percentages of carbs, fat, and protein at the beginning and at the end of the study. In contrast, by the second week of the experiment, the 5-HTP group was eating an average of 67 fewer grams of carbohydrates a day (the amount in 2½ cups of sugary breakfast cereal), and 12 fewer grams of fat (the amount in an ounce of cashews). In other words, 75 percent of their calorie-cutting was from carbs!

Shedding 2 pounds per week. The placebo group didn't lose any weight over the two weeks. The 5-HTP group lost an average of 4.6 pounds—or more than 2 pounds a week.

Low L-tryptophan. And—confirming the researchers' hypothesis—at the start of the study, the diabetics had much lower levels of L-tryptophan available to be converted into serotonin in the brain. (They didn't take this measurement at the end of the study.)

Improved diabetic parameters. The researchers also noted that the diabetics getting 5-HTP had lower blood sugar levels, lower insulin levels, and lower levels of *glycosolated hemoglobin* (the percentage of red blood cells in the blood with blood sugar attached), a measurement used to indicate the severity of diabetes.

Their conclusions?

Type 2 diabetics have lower levels of L-tryptophan available to their brains, perhaps leading them to eat too many calories and too many carbs.

Giving 5-HTP to diabetics helps them cut their calorie and carbohydrate intake, and also helps them lose weight.

Perhaps, says Dr. Rossi-Fanelli, 5-HTP should be a standard therapy for diabetics, helping them achieve better blood sugar levels—and therefore delaying major complications, like heart disease and stroke, kidney disease, blindness, and severe foot and leg problems, leading to amputation.

Are there other health problems 5-HTP might help improve or solve? Quite a few.

5-HTP FOR DEPRESSION, PAIN RELIEF, HOT FLASHES, AND MORE

Boosting serotonin levels can do a lot more than satisfy your appetite and cut your craving for carbs. Research shows that 5-HTP may help . . .

Depression. Over one hundred studies have looked at 5-HTP (or L-tryptophan) to relieve depression. In 2002, a review of the studies on depression and 5-HTP by Australian researchers concluded that 5-HTP is definitely "better than a placebo" in relieving depression. Much better, says Dr. Murray.

"Results of dozens of scientific studies have convinced me that 5-HTP is far superior to all types of prescription and antidepressant drugs— even the newer ones—for depression," he told us. He cites several advantages to 5-HTP in treating depression: the speed at which it works (for most patients, within two weeks of starting therapy, compared to four to six weeks for prescription drugs); the fact that it frequently works where other therapies don't (therapy-resistant depression); and the lack of side effects.

Interferon-induced depression. The drug interferon-alpha (IFN) is frequently prescribed to treat cancer and hepatitis C. Unfortunately, about one-third of the people who get it develop severe depression—and antidepressant drugs effectively treat only about 60 to 70 percent of those cases. Doctors at the Mood Disorders Research Center in Portland, Oregon, think that a combination of SSRIs *and* 5-HTP is the best treatment.

"We hypothesize that SSRIs are not fully effective because they affect only serotonin reuptake, not serotonin synthesis, and that effective treatment must address both uptake and synthesis," they write in the journal

Medical Hypothesis. In other words, antidepressant drugs help keep serotonin in the brain—but, unlike 5-HTP, they don't create additional serotonin in the body.

"5-HTP effectively increases central nervous system synthesis of serotonin," they continue, and recommend the drug *and* supplement treatment for anyone who becomes depressed after treatment with interferon.

Panic attacks and generalized anxiety disorder (GAD). A panic attack is anxiety or fear triggered for no obvious reason, accompanied by symptoms like shortness of breath, racing heart, trembling, and sweating.

Some degree of anxiety now and then is natural. But excessive anxiety— a constant, worried feeling for months at a time, perhaps accompanied by physical symptoms like dry mouth, clammy hands, stomachaches, and heart palpitations—is a clinically defined problem, called *generalized anxiety disorder*. And there are several other types of anxiety disorders, such as post-traumatic stress syndrome, obsessive–compulsive disorder, and social phobia, or shyness. All in all, some 19 million Americans suffer from a panic or anxiety disorder; 5-HTP might help.

In a study by Dutch doctors, patients suffering from anxiety were given either 5-HTP or an anti-anxiety drug. Those taking 5-HTP had a "moderate reduction" in their anxiety symptoms.

In another study from Holland, doctors gave patients suffering from panic disorder either 5-HTP or a placebo, and then induced panic attacks (with carbon dioxide, which causes shortness of breath). "5-HTP significantly reduced the reaction to the panic challenge in the panic disorder patients, regarding subjective anxiety, panic symptom score, and number of panic attacks," they write in the December 30, 2002 issue of *Psychiatry Research*.

Night terrors in children. Doctors at the Center for Pediatric Sleep Disorders at the University of Rome gave 5-HTP or a placebo to forty-five children with "night terrors"—a sudden arousal from sleep, with a piercing scream or cry, racing heart, fast breathing, and feelings of intense fear. Night terrors afflict children between the ages of four and twelve and can occur as infrequently as once per month or as frequently as every night.

After one month of taking 5-HTP at bedtime, 93 percent of children had a positive response. After six months, 84 percent were free of night terrors. "5-HTP is able to modulate the arousal level in children and induce a long-term improvement of sleep terrors," wrote the researchers in the *European Journal of Pediatrics* in 2004.

Tension and migraine headaches. Seven studies have shown positive results using 5-HTP to control migraines and tension headaches. In a study of 124 people, reported in *European Neurology*, 600 mg of 5-HTP daily either prevented or decreased the number of migraines in 75 percent of the people taking the supplement. And in a study of forty-eight elementary and junior high school students, published in *Drugs Under Experimental and Clinical Research*, 5-HTP decreased the frequency of tension headaches by 70 percent.

Fibromyalgia. In this mysterious disease, the sufferer (a woman, in three out of four cases) may have painful "tender points" in muscles all over her body, morning stiffness, insomnia, severe fatigue, and anxiety. (The condition is very similar to chronic fatigue syndrome, and some experts consider them the same problem.) Approximately 16 million Americans suffer from fibromyalgia. And 5-HTP can help treat it.

For ninety days, doctors in Italy gave 100 mg of 5-HTP three times a day to fifty people with fibromyalgia. In nearly half the patients, every symptom improved: tender points, severity of pain, sleep, fatigue, and anxiety. "5-HTP is effective in improving the symptoms of fibromyalgia," the researchers concluded, in the *Journal of International Medical Research*.

Hot flashes. Researchers at the Southwest College of Naturopathic Medicine, writing in *Alternative Medicine Review* in September 2005, theorize that 5-HTP could help reduce hot flashes and may be a particularly good nonhormonal therapy in postmenopausal women with a history of breast cancer or who are at a high risk for the disease. "Increased serotonin levels may have the ability to decrease hot flashes in a mechanism similar to that of SSRIs, without the risk of breast cell stimulation," they write.

Insomnia. "Several clinical studies have shown 5-HTP to produce good results in promoting and maintaining sleep in normal subjects as well as those experiencing insomnia," says Dr. Murray.

5-HTP is a more powerful antioxidant than vitamin C. Antioxidants like vitamin C improve health by fighting *free radicals*, molecules that damage cells, perhaps speeding aging and playing a role in heart disease and cancer. Scientists in Germany, writing in the *Journal of Pineal Research* in 2005, reported a study in which 5-HTP was seven times more powerful in defusing free radical molecules than vitamin C.

IS 5-HTP SAFE TO TAKE?

5-HTP supplements are made from the seeds of *Griffonia simplicifolia*, a plant naturally rich in the amino acid. Sounds innocent enough. But given what happened with L-tryptophan, maybe you're thinking twice about taking L-tryptophan's close biochemical relative. Sure, it was proven that the problem that killed more than forty people *wasn't* L-tryptophan but a contaminant in the supplements, generated by one manufacturer. Still, the fact that L-tryptophan supplements killed people might give you pause. And you wouldn't be alone.

Over the years, various scientists have looked closely at the relationship of L-tryptophan and 5-HTP—and subsequently questioned the safety of 5-HTP. Let's take a close look at their findings.

Was It EMS?

In 1994 there was a report in the *Journal of Rheumatology* describing the case of a Canadian mother of two infants (thirty-three months and thirteen months) who were give 5-HTP and a drug (L-dopa/cardidopa) to treat an inherited genetic disease of L-tryptophan metabolism. Although the mother never took 5-HTP, she handled the pills. And she developed an illness that had some symptoms similar to EMS, including muscle soreness and high eosinophil counts. Although it was never proven that she had EMS, it was concluded she *might* have had it.

Peak X

Scientists performed three sophisticated analytical tests on the 5-HTP taken by the Canadian woman's children: high-performance liquid chromatography (a technique used in analytic chemistry to separate a mixture into its component parts); mass spectrometry (a technique used to analyze molecules); and capillary electrophoresis (another method used to separate out components). They reported the chromatograph showed an impurity, which they dubbed "Peak X." However, neither of the other analytical methods spotted Peak X, and a later and more careful examination of the chromatographs showed no clear evidence of a "peak" of impurity.

In 1998, scientists at the Mayo Clinic also claimed to have found Peak X in 5-HTP. However, the same scientists later identified another compound as Peak X, and hypothesized (without any evidence) that Peak X might be *several* impurities.

In short, the presence of Peak X has *never* been scientifically established.

But manufacturers of 5-HTP now screen for it, to be certain that their products are free of "Peak X" as defined by the FDA.

Putting Facts Before Fears

Yesu Das, PhD, a colleague of Dr. Preuss, closely analyzed several samples of 5-HTP, finding no impurities. In fact, he concluded that "Peak X" wasn't an impurity at all, but an "artifact" produced by the analysis process itself. In an article on the safety of 5-HTP, published in *Toxicology Letter* in 2004, Dr. Das, Dr. Preuss, and two other colleagues from Creighton University discuss the almost zero likelihood that 5-HTP causes EMS:

> The primary cause of the widespread EMS was, and still is, attributed to contamination of a single source of product. In contrast, 5-HTP is produced by extraction from a plant source. Although this makes it highly unlikely that 5-HTP would contain a contaminant similar to L-tryptophan, the perception still exists. Despite the lack of solid cases of EMS-related disorders in recent years, there are still attempts to link intake of 5-HTP with this disorder. Suffice it to say that one must review in more detail the historical background of L-tryptophan toxicity and the validity of the concerns raised on 5-HTP in order to make valid judgments on the safety of 5-HTP and to put facts before fears.

Put facts before fears—and the fact is, 5-HTP is safe.

"In summary," write Dr. Preuss and his colleagues, "there is a dearth of evidence to implicate 5-HTP as a cause of any illness, especially EMS or its related disorders."

The Serotonin Syndrome

The right amount of serotonin does a body good. But get too much in your system, and you might become agitated and confused (even delirious), with a racing heartbeat, spikes in blood pressure, and heavy sweating. *Theoretically*, that could happen if you were taking SSRIs *and* 5-HTP.

"5-HTP shouldn't be used by people taking antidepressant drugs except under close medical supervision," says Dr. Murray.

He also says people taking the antimigraine drug methysergide (Sansert) or the antihistamine cyproheptadine (Periactin)—drugs that work by blocking serotonin—shouldn't take 5-HTP.

5-HTP OR SEROTONIN-BOOSTING PRESCRIPTION ANTI-OBESITY DRUGS: WHICH IS THE BETTER CHOICE?

There are several new serotonin-boosting prescription medications being tested for their effectiveness in weight loss in animal or clinical trials. Once on the market, will they be a better choice than 5-HTP?

"I am wary of using serotonin-boosting prescription drugs for weight loss," says Michael Murray, ND.

"Remember," he told us, "that in 1997, the popular weight-loss drug Redux and its chemical cousin, fenfluramine, part of the 'fen-phen' combination, were taken off the market based on a study showing that these drugs may have caused permanent damage to heart valves in as many as one-third of the people who took them. There is no evidence that 5-HTP produces these types of effects. Unlike Redux, 5-HTP does not raise blood serotonin levels to a significant degree, nor does it block the reuptake of serotonin in the brain. In short, it does not disrupt the normal process of serotonin release, reabsorption, and elimination from the body.

"5-HTP is not a synthetic drug. It is an amino acid, produced naturally by your body's metabolism. I think 5-HTP is and always will be the far superior choice for helping to boost serotonin levels as a way to aid in weight loss."

Not to Worry, Says Dr. Murray

Dr. Murray—who has given 5-HTP to literally hundreds of his patients—isn't concerned about the safety of the supplement. "There have been no reports of a single person developing EMS from 5-HTP, despite its popularity," he told us.

Evidence that uncontaminated 5-HTP does not cause EMS is also provided by researchers who have been using 5-HTP for over thirty years, as well as by researchers at the National Institutes of Health studying the effects of uncontaminated 5-HTP on various metabolic conditions.

To be on the safe side, however, Dr. Murray recommends that anyone regularly taking 5-HTP be monitored every six months with a eosinophil determination, which is part of a standard blood test known as a complete blood count (CBC).

He also says pregnant or lactating women should not take 5-HTP. Nor should people with Parkinson's disease (because it could interfere with drugs used to control levels of dopamine, a neurotransmitter). And people with scleroderma, a disease of connective tissue linked to a defect in L-tryptophan metabolism, should avoid the supplement.

MAXIMIZING 5-HTP FOR WEIGHT LOSS

For weight loss, Dr. Murray recommends 50 mg of 5-HTP, three times a day, twenty minutes before a meal.

What about the nausea experienced by some people when they take 5-HTP? After all, that's definitely *not* the way you want 5-HTP to help you stop overeating!

"I think it's quite critical that the capsules of 5-HTP be *enteric-coated*—coated in a way that prevents their being broken down in the stomach," says Dr. Murray. "Without enteric coating, 5-HTP almost always produces nausea," he says. "With enteric coating, this side effect rarely occurs."

Okay, you take 5-HTP with enteric coating—but how do you know it's working?

"If 5-HTP is the right approach, it will usually be obvious in many ways," says Dr. Murray. "Feeling less stressed, happier, and more in control are typical experiences." And, of course, you should start eating less. "In weight-loss studies, 5-HTP didn't reduce appetite, but it substantially increased *satiety*," says Dr. Murray. "In other words, don't expect 5-HTP to curb your appetite, but it should reduce the amount of food you require to feel full."

What should you do if you feel 5-HTP *isn't* working?

"After two weeks of use, you can increase the amount to 100 mg, three times a day," says Dr. Murray. But, we asked him, didn't the studies conducted by Dr. Rossi-Fanelli use a lot more 5-HTP—as much as 900 mg a day?

SUPPLEMENT SUPPORTER

JULIA ROSS, MA

www.dietcure.com, www.moodcure.com

Author, *The Diet Cure* and *The Mood Cure*; director, Recovery Systems Clinic, Mill Valley, California

In *The Diet Cure*, Julia Ross describes the eight (often overlooked) factors that cause overweight, either singly or in combination: brain chemistry imbalances; low-calorie dieting; unstable blood sugar; low thyroid function; addictions to food you're allergic to; hormonal havoc; yeast overgrowth; and fatty acid deficiency.

For imbalances in brain chemistry (which, she says, can cause carbohydrate cravings), she recommends amino acid supplements—including the amino acid discussed in this chapter: 5-HTP.

"Brain chemicals like serotonin fuel the brain's appetite-regulating sites," she told us. "If you're deficient in serotonin, you'll struggle with cravings for carbohydrates, which metabolize in such a way as to briefly boost serotonin in the brain."

And, she adds, food cravings are *the most common problem* for people struggling with weight. And the most common *time* for these cravings is in the afternoon and evening, when serotonin levels fall.

"Whenever sunlight diminishes, serotonin drops—and serotonin is a natural appetite normalizer *and* antidepressant," says Ross. "The solution: increase serotonin levels in the brain, in order to turn off food cravings and emotional overeating. One excellent way to do that: take the serotonin-boosting amino acid 5-HTP. People notice—even within ten minutes of getting the right dose—that their cravings end and their negative moods dissipate. So this supplement is terribly important for our obesity epidemic *and* our depression epidemic."

Ross recommends starting with 50 to 100 mg of 5-HTP, in the late afternoon, before the craving for sweets or starches kicks in. "For many people, that's all they need," she says.

"Yes, they did," said Dr. Murray. "But my own experience is that if 5-HTP is going to work for you, it's going to work just as well at 100 mg, three times a day, as at 300 mg three times a day."

And that's the level Dr. Preuss endorses. It's the lower level of intake, and therefore most likely to be safe.

Dr. Murray urges people to use "well-respected health-food store brands of 5-HTP" that are enteric-coated. Such brands include: Natural Factors, Nature's Way, Now, and Solaray.

9

Trying to Solve the Prickly Problem of Appetite

- ## Cacti: Caralluma and Hoodia

"I'm hungry."

That's a pretty simple statement. You've said it—and your body has felt it—thousands of times. In fact, maybe you're feeling hungry right now. Hey, no problem. Go ahead and visit the kitchen for a healthy snack. We'll be here when you get back.

When you're hungry, you eat. Not too complicated, right?

But what's *really* happening when you feel hungry—when you have an appetite? How is your stomach communicating with your brain? What hormones is your endocrine system pumping out? And is there a way to *control* appetite—to turn it down? (Maybe even *off*?) Or is hunger simply a natural force, like the weather, that can't be altered, slowed, or stopped?

Obviously, those are important questions to answer for people who want to lose weight—and for the scientists who want to help them.

You might think figuring out how appetite works wouldn't be all that hard. Like we said, what could be more straightforward than the urge to eat? But the science of appetite isn't simple. There's a monthly scientific journal called *Appetite*, devoted to nothing but the study of the phenomenon. And researchers all over the world continue to investigate appetite, discovering (and debating) new facts about how it works.

We're making such a big fuss over appetite because this chapter is about two plants that are reported to work by affecting it—plants that *might* help you lose weight by helping you feel a lot less hungry. (We emphasized the *might* in that last sentence—as in maybe, possibly, potentially—because the supplements we're discussing in this chapter don't have enough strong scientific evidence to support them. But we're telling you about them because they're intriguing, and because a lot of dieters take them.)

Meet the cacti, *caralluma fimbriata* and *hoodia gordonii*.

Cacti are the camels of the plant world. They've adapted to survive in sandy, nutrient-poor soil, on very little water. So perhaps it's not all that surprising that these two plants contain unique molecules that might affect hunger, temporarily reducing it. How do they do that? To find out, let's delve a little deeper into the Science of Hungerology . . .

THE MYSTERY OF APPETITE

The understanding of appetite took a giant leap (or bite) forward in 1994. That was the year scientists at Rockefeller University in New York City discovered the hormone *leptin*. Produced by fat cells, leptin sends messages to cells in the hypothalamus, the part of the brain that maintains the body's status quo, or what scientists call *homeostasis*.

Too hot? Your hypothalamus tells the body to cool down. Tired? Your hypothalamus tells the body to go to sleep. Thirsty? Drink up, says your hypothalamus. The hypothalamus gets its information from receptors in the organ itself (like *thermoreceptors*, to monitor temperature) and from signals relayed to it by the optic nerve, spinal cord, brainstem, and other areas. Leptin is one of those signals: it tells the hypothalamus about energy levels in the body, thereby turning on or turning off brain cells that contain the hormones and amino acids that help regulate appetite.

When you need (or don't need) more food, your hypothalamus knows. And when you *do* need more food, it tells you that you're hungry.

After the discovery of leptin, there was a flurry of research into appetite. And scientists soon began to realize that hunger *is* a lot like the weather—a complex system of causes and effects, of forces and feedback, of interactions and influences, with the brain, nervous system, digestive tract, and various hormones all playing their part. But they also figured out that the master controller of the entire process is . . . the hypothalamus.

HYPOTHALAMUS: HUNGER CENTRAL

The name is strange but logical: the hypothalamus is under (hypo) the thalamus, the part of the brain that relays messages to the cerebral cortex. The hypothalamus is shaped like a cone, with a tubular tip connected to the pituitary gland, the "master" gland of the hormonal system. As we explained above, the hypothalamus sends out messages that keep the body balanced. It does this in two ways.

It sends messages to the autonomic nervous system—so named because it controls "autonomous" functions that run without conscious control, like heart rate, blood pressure, body temperature, and digestion.

And it sends messages to the pituitary gland to secrete hormones that, in turn, direct the activity of the entire hormonal system, which pumps out hormones like insulin (to balance blood sugar) and adrenaline (to energize the body when there's a challenge or threat).

Yes, scientists have figured out that the hypothalamus is the master regulator of appetite. But they haven't quite figured out *how* it does that. (Leptin is only one piece of the puzzle.) And this is where caralluma and hoodia come in. Both of them contain *glycosides*, biochemicals that affect the hunger mechanisms of the hypothalamus. And scientific studies of how these glycosides affect the hypothalamus may reveal more about how the brain regulates appetite.

GLYCOSIDES—THEY'RE ON YOUR SIDE

Glycosides are molecules in plants. Chemically speaking, they're a sugar (carbohydrate) bonded to a non-sugar by carbon atoms.

There are lots of different glycosides. Hoodia is rich in *steroidal glycosides* (which are used to treat heart disease, in the drug digitalis). Caralluma is rich in *pregnane glycosides* (which are also found in HCA supplements discussed in Chapter 3). When it comes to controlling hunger, both of these glycosides might be on your side. Because, as we said a moment ago, scientists theorize that both of them affect the hypothalamus so that your brain tells you that you're *not* hungry.

Hyper-Energy for the Hypothalamus

Led by David B. MacLean, MD, researchers in the Division of Endocrinology at Brown University, in Rhode Island, conducted a series of studies on P57, an extract of the steroidal glycosides in hoodia. Here's what they found.

Energy in the hypothalamus—increased. When they injected P57 into the hypothalamic cells of rat brains, it boosted by 50 to 150 percent the cellular level of ATP (adenosine triphosphate, a molecule that is the fundamental form of energy for chemical reactions in the body).

Low brain energy from dieting—prevented. The researchers also found that when animals were put on a low-calorie diet, ATP levels in hypothalamus cells dropped—but the drop was subsequently prevented by injections of P57.

Food intake—lowered. And the researchers found that P57 reduced food intake in rats by 40 to 60 percent.

A New Theory of Hunger

Based on their findings, the scientists speculate that ATP levels in the brain reflect energy levels in the body—that when the hypothalamus "senses" ATP levels are low, it triggers brain cells and hormones to make an announcement to the body: "You're hungry!" When ATP is high, the hypothalamus doesn't trigger those cells and hormones. Since the glycosides in the hoodia extract increased ATP in hypothalamic cells, you could say they "tricked" the brain into not sending hunger messages.

Dr. Preuss and other researchers theorize that the pregnane glycosides in caralluma also affect hunger mechanisms in the hypothalamus.

According to this theory, if you're dieting, the glycosides from caralluma or hoodia might energize your hypothalamus so that it doesn't send out hunger signals.

Let's look at those two cacti, one by one.

CARALLUMA: THE "FAMINE FOOD" THAT MIGHT HELP STOP HUNGER

Okay, it's time to tell you: although caralluma and hoodia are commonly referred to as cacti, they're actually *succulents*, a water-storing plant that grows in hot and dry climates. The succulent *caralluma fimbriata* grows in Africa, Arabia, southern Europe, and Afghanistan.

But it's in India where caralluma is perhaps best known. It grows just about everywhere—in cities and towns, as a roadside shrub, as a boundary marker in gardens. But people in India don't just cultivate caralluma as an ornamental plant. They also eat it.

In the Kolli Hills of South India, it's eaten like a vegetable. In the arid regions of Andhra Pradesh, in southeast India, it's used in pickles and chutney. And in western India, caralluma has been eaten for thousands of years . . . when there isn't much else to eat. It's listed as a "famine food" in the Indian Health Ministry's comprehensive compilation of medicinal plants—a food that has helped people who don't have enough to eat feel a little less hungry.

Well, you're probably not too worried about the next famine. But if caralluma can reduce hunger when there's very little food around, maybe it can do the same when there's too much food around. Two scientific studies on overweight people and caralluma explored exactly that issue.

A Study in India

A study on caralluma and weight loss was conducted by Dr. A.V. Kurpad and his colleagues at St. John's Medical College in Bangalore, India, and reported at the 18th International Congress of Nutrition, in September 2005.

Dr. Kurpad used an herbal extract of the pregnane glycosides of caralluma—the same amount of glycosides you'd get if you ate a little more than 3 ounces a day of the cactus.

He studied fifty overweight people, with an average BMI (body mass index, a measure of overweight) of 26 or more. For eight weeks, twenty-five people received caralluma and twenty-five a placebo. They weren't asked to cut calories, but they were instructed to walk thirty minutes in the morning and again in the evening.

The results were encouraging.

Weight loss—42 percent more. Those taking caralluma lost 4.3 pounds. Those getting the placebo lost 2.5.

BMI reduction—30 percent greater. Those taking caralluma lost a full point from their BMI. Those taking the placebo lost 0.7.

Thinner waists and hips. The waistlines and hips of those on caralluma firmed up quite a bit. The measurements of those on the placebo didn't budge.

More fat loss. The caralluma group lost a lot more fat than the placebo group. (Dr. Preuss thinks the same glycosides that affect the hypothalamus may also block an enzyme that sparks your body's fat-making machinery.)

Less hunger. And, most important, the people taking caralluma reported feeling a lot less hungry than those on the placebo.

A Study in California

A second study on a caralluma extract was conducted by Ronald Lawrence, MD, and his colleagues at the Western Geriatric Institute in Los Angeles,

California, and reported at the 12th Annual World Congress on Anti-Aging Medicine, in 2004.

It lasted one month and looked at twenty-six overweight people— seventeen women and nine men, thirty-one to seventy-three years old. Nineteen took caralluma and seven a placebo. They were told not to change their eating or exercise habits during the study. The results:

Nine pounds lost in one month. Fifteen people on caralluma lost weight. (On average, the placebo group gained a little weight.) Eleven of those lost 6 pounds or more, with the highest loss at 9 pounds. Four others lost 1 to 2 pounds. The other four didn't lose any weight. There was almost no weight loss in the placebo group.

Lower body mass. The BMI of the caralluma group went from an average of 30.7 to 28.9. The placebo group, from 26.6 to 26.7.

Slimmer waists. Thirteen of the nineteen people on caralluma had a waist reduction of half an inch to 3 inches. As for hips: the caralluma group lost an average 1.82 inches, the placebo group 0.08.

"Further studies of this interesting succulent are recommended," writes Dr. Lawrence. (A conclusion Dr. Preuss agrees with: the findings on caralluma are positive—and preliminary.)

Dr. Lawrence also comments on the safety of caralluma: "Of great significance is the lack of toxicity and lack of side effects produced by caralluma. This was noted on the original Indian study . . . and is verified by us."

Safe to Take

There's other evidence that caralluma is safe.

No side effects in studies. In both studies, there were no more side effects among those who took caralluma than among the placebo group.

NATURAL FAT-LOSS PHARMACY SUCCESS STORY

Putting the Brakes on Late-Night Snacking

Mitch L. is a hard-driving executive at a food company in southern Florida.

At six foot three and 205 pounds, he's got a BMI of 25.3—which government officials would say means he's *slightly* overweight. Mitch disagrees.

"Hey," Mitch joked with us, "I work out in the gym a couple of times a week. Those pounds are pure muscle!"

In other words, Mitch *isn't* overweight, even slightly. But he was a little worried about getting that way.

"Late-night snacking is one of my weaknesses," he says. "I find myself pacing in the kitchen, with this overwhelming need to eat, even though I'm not hungry. And you know what they say: 'After eight, gain weight.' "

Mitch read about caralluma and its hunger-suppressing powers and decided to take a pill with dinner. "The results were amazing," he says. "I found that I wasn't even interested in food after dinner. My late-night snacking problem was solved."

Mitch was so enthusiastic about the way caralluma worked that he recommended it to his friends Jeff and Kathy W., a married couple in their mid-forties who eat out a lot and find it hard to resist the huge, yummy-looking portions.

"Caralluma has helped them, too," says Mitch. "They find they're just not as hungry at mealtime. They're eating less—and both of them have lost a pants size. Jeff and Kathy are the kind of people who are skeptics about everything. But now they tell everybody they know about caralluma!"

No changes in blood chemistry. The Indian researchers measured blood chemistry, and there were no significant changes among those taking caralluma—no major ups or downs in the sixteen different measurements, no indication the supplement was hurting the body in any way.

It's in the food supply. In India, people have eaten caralluma for thousands of years—strong evidence for its safety.

The supplement is widely used. And the supplement itself has been on the market for a number of years, without any reports of negative side effects.

"I believe that *Caralluma fimbriata* is safe to consume at recommended doses," concluded Dr. Preuss, in a paper he wrote on the safety of the plant and its extract.

Caralluma-Containing Products

If you decide to take caralluma, look for products that contain *Slimaluma*, the standardized extract of caralluma that was used in the clinical studies conducted in India and the U.S. As we went to press, the only product on the market containing only Slimaluma was GenaSlim, from Country Life. There are a few other supplements that contain Slimaluma—but, in each case, the ingredient is combined with one or more other ingredients that have not been proven to aid weight loss. As more Slimaluma-containing supplements enter the market, look for those that contain *only* (or at least *mostly*) Slimaluma, rather than combinations including the herb and unproven ingredients.

The recommended daily dosage on the GenaSlim label is the same as that used in the clinical study from India that helped people lose weight: 625 milligrams (mg), three times a day, one hour before meals. If you take GenaSlim, follow that recommendation.

HOODIA—OR HOODWINKED?

Google "hoodia" and surf a few sites. You'll immediately find yourself riding the waves of the real and the fake . . .

"Authentic Hoodia Gordonii!"

"Which really work?"

"Hoodia rip-offs—read this before you buy!"

"Don't be fooled by those cheap imitators!"

"Real Hoodia fast!"

"Many claim to have Hoodia Gordonii but in reality what they are offering you . . ."

Yes, when you enter the helter-skelter world of hoodia, you enter the world of controversy, conflict, claims, counterclaims—and (for the uninitiated) nearly complete confusion! To help you understand why that's so, we need to fill you in on a little hoodia history, starting about 20,000 years ago . . .

Bushmen with Hunger Pangs

Imagine you're a San, or Bushman, in the Kalahari Desert of southern Africa—a tribesperson in the world's oldest indigenous culture. On hunting and gathering trips in this barren wilderness, you're likely to travel for days without access to food and water. But Nature provides a solution. A six-foot-high, green, prickly, and bitter-tasting plant you call *Xhoba*. Throughout your journey, you slice off the cucumber-shaped stalks, eat the milky centers . . . and move on, without hunger or thirst.

Modern-day scientists call this unusual plant *hoodia gordonii*.

The P57 Patent

In the mid-sixties, scientists in South Africa began to study hoodia, as part of a project on edible wild plants that investigated several hundred species. Among their findings: when they fed hoodia to lab animals, the animals ate less and lost weight.

By 1997, they had isolated its active ingredient, which they dubbed P57 (because it was the 57th compound from the plant they'd tested).

A few years later, the Council for Scientific and Industrial Research (CSIR) granted the patent for P57 to Phytopharm, a British pharmaceutical company, which subsequently tested it on people in a small study, conducted in 2001. (We'll tell you about the results of that study in a moment.)

Phytopharm then sold the rights to P57 to Pfizer, the multinational drug company, which in 2003 decided not to try to formulate and market a synthetic form of the extract.

(In the midst of all this, the Bushmen, represented by a South African lawyer, entered into negotiations with the CSIR, demanding—and getting—a percentage of the sales of P57.)

In 2004, the rights to P57 were sold to Unilever (we warned you the world of hoodia is complicated!), another multinational company, specializing in foods (Slim-Fast, Hellmann's, Lipton) and personal care (Dove, Lux, Ponds). Industry reports suggest that Unilever may incorporate P57 into their Slim-Fast brand, with products scheduled to hit the market in 2008.

If Unilever has the patent to the extract, what's *in* the hoodia being sold on the shelves? Few really know (though many claim they do).

Hoodia Becomes Famous

In 2004, the show *60 Minutes* did a feature on hoodia, championing the rights of the San—and also showing Lesley Stahl eating a bit of hoodia and then claiming she didn't feel hungry the rest of the day. "I'd have to say it did work," Stahl declared.

Hoodia quickly became a weight-loss celebrity. And hoodia supplements—*lots* of hoodia supplements—began appearing.

Many Web sites will tell you about the bogus nature of these supplements, saying they contain hoodia grown in Mexico or China and not the Kalahari Desert . . . use a hoodia species that's not gordonii . . . use the wrong part of the plant . . . use only the seeds . . . or simply don't contain any hoodia at all. And then they sell you *their* supplement, which they claim is the only one on the market that *really* contains hoodia.

Other sites assert that buying an authentic hoodia supplement is only a little less complicated than paying taxes—that any *real* hoodia must be accompanied with a C.I.T.E.S. certificate (Convention on International Trade in Endangered Species of Wild Fauna and Flora), a Classification II-W (not any other classification, mind you), an FDA registration number, a USDA permit to export, and a Cape Nature Export Certificate.

Well, maybe hoodia works because in doing the background check on the brand you want to take you simply don't have time to eat!

Okay, that's not true.

There are a couple of very preliminary studies on animals and humans that show hoodia may have some promise.

STUDIES ON HOODIA

As with most nutritional research, the first studies were done on animals.

50 percent less fat. Lean and obese rats fed hoodia extract for several weeks had decreased food intake and weight loss. In some of the obese rats, body fat was reduced by 50 percent, compared to rats not getting hoodia.

Diabetes reversed. In an unpublished study (discussed by the researchers at Brown University, in their paper on P57), overweight, diabetic rats were given hoodia extract for eight weeks. The rats ate much less, and the diabetes was reversed.

Importantly, none of these studies showed any toxic reactions from taking hoodia.

One thousand fewer calories a day. There's been one clinical study on hoodia extract, conducted by Phytopharm, the company that sold the patent on hoodia extract to Pfizer and Unilever.

For two weeks, eighteen overweight people lived in a "metabolic unit"—a place where meals and activity are carefully controlled. In this case, the study participants were allowed to eat as much as they wanted. Nine took hoodia extract and nine took a placebo.

Over the two weeks, those taking hoodia extract spontaneously reduced their calorie intake by 1,000—from an average of 3,000 to an average of 2,000 a day.

On average the hoodia group lost about 4½ pounds and also had lower levels of blood fat (triglycerides) and blood sugar.

NATURAL FAT-LOSS PHARMACY
SUCCESS STORY

Can Seventy People All Be Wrong?

There's very little scientific evidence that hoodia works. But there are a lot of people who say it does.

In researching this chapter, we located seventy of them, after contacting Jason Odom, the owner of the Web site www.hoodiagordinii.com, who urged us to pass on his success story and the stories of more than sixty other people who have gleefully shared the good news of their weight loss, assisted by hoodia. (Jeff is quick to point out that he doesn't sell hoodia at his site.) A thirty-nine-year-old, he claims to have lost 30 pounds in eighty-nine days, taking approximately 3,000 to 5,000 mg of hoodia a day. (He varied his dosage, depending on how hungry he felt.) We couldn't really say his approach was healthy. On Day 7 of his weight-loss journey, he wrote in his diary, "Feeling better until I drank a stiff drink and took 750 mg of hoodia at the same time on an empty stomach. WOW, dizzy and buzzed like crazy. Had to lay down. Didn't eat breakfast or lunch. Slept through dinner. DON'T drink and take hoodia at the same time." (Good advice.)

His tale of weight loss is followed by those of his sixty or so fellow hoodia lovers. Among them . . .

A twenty-six-year-old woman who went from 198 to 164 pounds taking 2,250 mg a day. "Had little to no appetite," she remarks.

A sixty-one-year-old woman who went from 169 to 148 pounds, losing 1.5 to 2 pounds a week on a low-carb diet and thirty minutes or more of exercise a day. She took a 750 mg dosage before leaving for work. Weight loss, she says, "is actually starting to be fun!"

A forty-five-year-old man who was extremely obese, at 388 pounds, and who has lost 82 pounds, taking 1,900 mg a day. "This really works," he says. "It really reduced my dependency on that 'full' feeling."

If all that "really" is for real, then these anecdotes about hoodia—and dozens more like them—are certainly intriguing.

So, Is There Any Real Hoodia Out There?

There's an independent and reliable organization that tests supplements to see if they contain what they claim they do: ConsumerLab.com, run by Todd Cooperman, MD.

In October 2005, ConsumerLab took a look at hoodia supplements—
and decided not to test them (in contrast to over seventy products and product categories they have tested, from acidophilus to zinc), saying,

> There is presently no scientific standard for assessing the quality of
> hoodia as an ingredient, although attempts are being made to charac-
> terize its components. The quality of hoodia supplements, therefore,
> remains largely uncertain. Once there is better characterization,
> ConsumerLab.com will likely purchase, test, and report on the qual-
> ity of marketed products.

And their conclusion about hoodia overall?

"Although tantalizing, the evidence for hoodia as a weight loss ingredient remains anecdotal and preliminary, as does evidence of its safety. It is
also uncertain which products on the market provide the authentic ingredient and whether they recommend an appropriate dose."

Ditto, said a spokesman for Unilever, speaking to the *New York Times*
in April 2005. They tested ten supplement brands to see if any contained
significant quantities of P57. Two had none. Four had small amounts. Four
had significant amounts.

Ditto, says Alkemists Pharmaceuticals, Inc., a company in Cosa Mesa,
California.

They routinely test batches of hoodia for authenticity, using three
highly sophisticated analysis techniques: digital photo-microscopy (DPM),
high-performance thin-layer chromatography (HPTLC), and high-
performance liquid chromatography (HPLC).

They, too, have found that many well-advertised products are bogus.
But, like Unilver, they found some hoodia products are for real. And
they've given their Certificate of Analysis to several products on the
market.

If you're going to buy and use hoodia, look for that certificate: a small
circular stamp (the certificate) with the name of Alkemists Pharmaceuticals.
Products verified to contain P57 by Alkemists include: Desert Burn; Etho
Africa Hoodia; King Hoodia; Hoodoba Pure; Hoodia Gordonii Trim Fast;

SUPPLEMENT SUPPORTER

FRED PESCATORE, MD

www.hamptonsdiet.com

Author, *The Hamptons Diet* and *The Hamptons Diet Cookbook*; president, AHCC Research Association; former associate medical director, Atkins Center

---

In the hallowed tradition of diet docs who hail from trendy, upscale locations like South Beach and Sonoma, Dr. Fred Pescatore advises you from the Hamptons—to eat like you lived by the Mediterranean. His diet includes lots of monounsaturated fats (with an emphasis on macadamia rather than olive oil), along with other "real foods" like vegetables, fish, lean meats, nuts, whole grains, and low-sugar fruits.

Dr. Pescatore also advises some of his patients to give the Hamptons Diet a helping hand with a weight-loss supplement from South . . . no, not Beach. South Africa.

"I've had good success with hoodia, in spite of all the seeming hype," he told us. "A sixty-four-year-old woman patient attributed her 40-pound weight loss to hoodia. She said she was able to lose weight for the first time in her life because her appetite was finally under control."

Dr. Pescatore also favors EGCG (green tea extract). "I put another patient of mine on EGCG who had never been able to lose weight. She was peri-menopausal, and the hormonal ups and downs of that time of life can make it very difficult to shed pounds. Her dose was 100 milligrams, three times a day. She had amazing success after adding that supplement to her regimen, and lost eighty-three pounds."

And, says Dr. Pescatore, *every* one of his overweight patients is asked to take a chromium supplement, which helps regulate blood sugar. "This supplement is a particular must for helping diabetics lose weight," he adds. "Without it, they typically can't achieve the weight-loss success they want to achieve."

He cites the case of a seventy-four-year-old woman who had uncontrolled diabetes, even though she was on three oral medications. "I put her on high-dose chromium—400 micrograms, three times a day—and was able to get her off two of those medications. She also started to lose weight. When I first saw her she weighed 210 pounds. Now she weighs 164."

Powerslim from Hoodia Products; Hoodia from Paradise Herbs; Hoodi-Thin; and Slimvivo Hoodia Gordonii.

Should you take any of those products?

Dr. Preuss says to wait.

Until there is a standard, reliable version of hoodia extract on the market, he thinks there are more reliable ways to reduce hunger, including HCA and 5-HTP.

PART VI

Muscle Builders

Make Exercise More Effective

- HMB (Hydroxy Methylbutyrate)
- BCAA (Branched-Chain Amino Acids)

Think for a second about the top-selling weight-loss books from the past couple of years. There's *Bob Greene's Total Body Makeover* and *Body for Life* and *The Ultimate New York Body Plan* and *8 Minutes in the Morning* and *Curves* and *Walk Away the Pounds* and . . . well, you get the idea. A lot of people *exercise* to lose weight. And they're literally moving in the right direction. (For more on why exercise is a must—particularly for weight maintenance—please see Chapter 14, Step Right Up to Weight Control.)

There are two nutritional supplements that might help you *stick* with your exercise program *and* improve its calorie-burning, body-firming results. They are:

- HMB (hydroxy methylbutyrate)

- BCAA (branched-chain amino acids)

But before we introduce you to these two exercise-assisting nutrients, you need to know two crucial facts about *what* they're assisting: your muscles.

Muscle Fact #1: Muscle tissue isn't static. Muscle is constantly being made, broken down, and remade. The building block of all that remodeling is *protein*. The protein/muscle equation is very simple:

- If your body makes more protein than it breaks down, you gain muscle.

- If your body makes less protein than it breaks down, you lose muscle.

Muscle Fact #2: Muscle is a metabolic powerhouse. The more muscle you have, the more calories you burn. That's because muscle is metabolically active. Someone with a lot of muscle burns 35 to 70 more calories a day than someone with a lot of fat!

Exercise, then, helps you lose weight in *two* ways. First, it incinerates calories. Second, it builds more calorie-burning muscle. But if you're exercising for weight loss, your muscles can run (or bike or walk or swim) into a couple of problems.

Soreness. Maybe you feel so sore after exercise that you lose your motivation to do it.

Injury. Maybe you hurt yourself during exercise, with a muscle sprain or strain, and subsequently can't do any more.

Protein erosion. Maybe there's a metabolic process going on in your body that you're not aware of: during exercise, muscle can burn its own protein for energy. This means that even though you're exercising, you're not making more muscle—and maybe you're even losing some.

If there were a way to exercise and *protect* your muscles so that you didn't get sore, hurt, or burn muscle for fuel . . . you'd be more likely to keep exercising, and keep maintaining and building muscle—and losing or maintaining weight.

Well, there is a way to protect your muscles. Two ways, in fact. HMB and BCAA. Let's look at them one by one.

HMB: HEAVY-DUTY MUSCLE BUILDING

HMB isn't an A-list nutrient. It's a *metabolite*, or breakdown product, of another nutrient: leucine, an amino acid. (Amino acids are the components of protein.) About 5 percent of the leucine in your diet becomes HMB. The biochemical dominoes fall like this . . .

In the liver, leucine becomes a *ketone* (a simple and very usable form of energy) called KIC. Then an enzyme (a protein that speeds up chemical reactions) goes to work on KIC, changing it into HMB. And as far as your muscles are concerned, HMB is ready to rumble.

Shielding and Strengthening Muscle

HMB has the ability to stop *proteolysis*, or the destruction of protein. In everyday terms, that means HMB can *increase* the protein that's made and *decrease* the protein that's destroyed. And as we mentioned earlier, that's a big deal for exercisers.

One of the ways exercise works to strengthen muscles is by naturally destroying the protein of muscle cells, causing the body to rebuild even more protein. In other words, exercise tears down and builds up, leading to bigger, stronger muscles. But sometimes the tearing down is more than the building up—leading to soreness, injury, and less than optimal gains in muscle size and strength. HMB protects muscles from some of that destruction, and then lends a hand in the rebuilding.

How does it do that? To find out, we talked to Steven L. Nissen, PhD, a professor at Iowa State University who, with his colleagues, has conducted more research on HMB than any other scientist.

Protecting Membranes

"Nobody knows for certain how HMB works, but we're fairly comfortable with our hypothesis: it supplies a building block that the muscle can't make enough of in stressful situations, like intense exercise," Dr. Nissen told us. You might be a little surprised to learn that the building block is . . . cholesterol, a fat with a bad reputation. Dr. Nissen explains:

> You can't build a muscle cell without cholesterol, which functions as a stabilizing component of the muscle membrane, or outer covering. Muscle is unique, however, in that it can't take cholesterol out of the blood and use it to make muscle—it's got to have the cholesterol *within* the cell. Normally, that's not a problem. But in situations where muscle cells are damaged—like heavy-duty exercise and aging—the body can't make enough cholesterol within the muscle to repair the harm. That's where HMB comes in. In the body, HMB is a must for manufacturing cholesterol. When you take HMB in sufficient quantities in supplemental form, you provide enough so that cholesterol can be made within damaged muscle cells. And that's the likely way that HMB protects, repairs, and strengthens muscles, and enhances muscle growth.

A Little Doesn't Go a Long Way

If your body produces HMB, why do you need a supplement?

Well, if you weigh 150 pounds or so, you produce about 0.2 to 0.4 grams a day—about ten times *less* than the 3 grams a day used in most of the studies that showed HMB can protect and build muscle.

And don't look for an HMBurger on the menu, to make up the difference. Even diets extremely high in protein can't deliver the amount of leucine necessary to generate a muscle-protecting level of HMB.

True, there are some foods that are richer in HMB than others. (Although even they don't supply a lot of the nutrient.) The two best sources are . . . alfalfa sprouts and catfish. Yum.

No, to get the HMB you need, you need a supplement. And supplements definitely can work.

BIGGER, STRONGER MUSCLES

Study after study shows that HMB can help build muscle size and strength, and help protect against soreness and possible injury.

Resistance Training—Turbocharged

One of the first and best studies on HMB and weight training (also called *resistance training*) was conducted by Dr. Nissen and his colleagues at Iowa State University, and reported in the *American Journal of Physiology* in 1996.

The study participants were forty-one healthy young men, aged nineteen to twenty-nine, who hadn't been lifting weights for at least three months before the study started.

First, the researchers divided the men into two groups. During the study, both groups ate a normal but nutrient-controlled diet, using entrées from Weight Watchers, Healthy Choice, and similar brands. One group, however, also got a protein supplement containing three times the recommended daily allowance (RDA) for protein. (Bodybuilding magazines and products often tout extra protein as a must for bigger muscles, and the researchers wanted to test this claim.)

Next, the researchers further divided each of these two groups into three subgroups with various levels of daily HMB intake, provided by a supplement: 0 grams (a placebo), 1.5 grams, or 3 grams.

At the beginning of the study, the researchers measured the men's muscle strength and body composition (percentage of muscle and fat).

To calculate breakdown of muscle protein the researchers also took weekly measurements of three biochemicals that show up in the blood or urine when muscle is being broken down by exercise: CK, LDH, and 3-MH, for you acronym lovers out there. And for the truly science-obsessed, who demand the name, the whole name, and nothing but the name: plasma creatine phosphokinase, lactate dehydrogenase, and urinary 3-methylhisti-dine, respectively.

The study lasted three weeks. During that time, the men lifted weights three times a week, using a combination of free weights (barbells) and weight machines (like Nautilus). They performed fourteen resistance exercises for the lower and upper body (bench press, calf raises, inclined sit-up, and the like).

The guys getting HMB got a real lift.

Leaner. The men getting 1.5 grams of HMB had *twice* the muscle gain of those getting the placebo. The guys getting 3 grams had *three times* the muscle gain.

Stronger. All the participants were lifting weights and they all got stronger. The placebo group got 8 percent stronger. The 1.5 gram HMB group got 13 percent stronger. The 3 gram HMB group got 18 percent stronger.

Hardier. When they started resistance training, the men getting the placebo went from 3 percent of muscle broken down per day to 6 percent. The 1.5 gram HMB group increased from 3 to 5.5 percent. The 3.0 gram HMB group increased from 3 to 4.5 percent. In other words, the more HMB they were taking, the more their muscles were protected.

No help from protein. The extra protein didn't help with muscle gain, muscle strength, or preventing muscle breakdown.

Dr. Nissen's conclusion, published in the *Journal of Applied Physiology*: "Supplementation with either 1.5 or 3 grams of HMB can partly prevent exercise-induced proteolysis [protein destruction] and/or muscle damage and result in larger gains in muscle function associated with resistance training."

NATURAL FAT-LOSS PHARMACY SUCCESS STORY

Two-Time World Bodybuilding Champion

Ben Tennessen is a thirty-one-year-old physical education teacher and strength coach at a high school in Wisconsin—and a world champion bodybuilder. He won the American competition of the Natural Bodybuilding Federation in 2004, and went on to win the world competition in 2004 and 2005. He's appeared several times on the cover of *Natural Bodybuilding and Fitness*. He's the current Arnold Schwarzenegger of the pumped-up professionals who won't touch a steroid with a ten-foot barbell.

Ben doesn't attribute his success in professional bodybuilding to HMB and BCAA. Those kudos, he says, go to his genetic gifts and to a super-rigorous training regimen. But in the elite world of professional bodybuilding, every little bit helps . . . and HMB and BCAA, he told us, have definitely made a difference.

"For HMB, I use the Advocare product Muscle Strength—and the results fit the name," says Ben. "I taper off quite a bit on my overall regimen of supplements during the off-season. But when I add HMB, within a week I can feel that I am much stronger in my workouts."

BCAA, he says, helps preserve muscle mass. "One of the keys to competitive edge in bodybuilding is to preserve muscle mass even in the midst of a calorie-restricted nutritional regimen that tries to eliminate practically every last ounce of body fat so that muscles look razor-sharp. On that kind of regimen, a lot of guys lose muscle in the final stages of getting ready for a show. But I never do. In fact, I get bigger. I attribute that to taking BCAA."

In the decade since this study was conducted, nearly a dozen other studies on HMB and weightlifting have shown similarly positive results.

That's great news for people starting a weightlifting regimen or any type of exercise.

If you take HMB, there's a very good possibility you'll see better results in strength gains, with less muscle loss from the stress of exercise. You'll be firmer, stronger—and maybe you'll be more inspired to *stick* with your routine, always the biggest challenge for the new exerciser. (And veterans, too!)

Less Soreness

In a study conducted by researchers at Kingston University in the UK, six men took either HMB (in combination with KIC, the HMB precursor) or a placebo for fourteen days. Then they performed a resistance exercise for the arms—a tough experimental exercise designed to induce muscle damage.

The men taking HMB/KIC had much less muscle soreness twenty-four hours after doing the exercise. Over the next three days, they also had lower levels of CK, better range of motion (another indication of less muscle damage), and less swelling (ditto).

The study was reported in the August 2005 issue of the *International Journal of Sport Nutrition and Exercise Metabolism.*

Running Without Getting Run-Down

In another study from Iowa State University, Dr. Nissen and his colleagues looked at long-distance runners. Runners putting in major mileage suffer a lot of muscle damage during and after their runs—so much so, they usually don't run as well in the days following a particularly long run.

The researchers looked at eight women and five men between the ages of twenty and fifty, all of whom ran at least thirty miles per week. They gave one group 3 grams of HMB a day and the other a placebo.

The researchers measured CK and LDH a few times during the study: at the beginning; after four weeks of supplementation with HMB; immediately after a very long run (twelve miles, including three miles of hills); and every day for four days after the long run.

HMB shielded the runners' muscles.

Let's look at the CK measurements in detail—so you can see just how strong that shield is. (Remember: CK is a reliable indicator of the degree of muscle breakdown.)

Right before the run, the HMB group's CK was 13 percent lower than that of the placebo group. (They'd already been taking HMB for four weeks.) Right after the run, it was 11 percent lower. One day after, it was 32 percent lower. Two days after, 33 percent lower. Three days after, 33 percent lower. Four days after, 11 percent lower. Less muscle destruction, before the run and after.

A similar (though not as numerically dramatic) trend was seen with LDH.

"These findings support the hypothesis that HMB supplementation helps prevent exercise-induced muscle damage," wrote Dr. Nissen, in the *Journal of Applied Physiology*.

HMB Works in the Young and the . . . Mature

Maybe you're reading this with reading glasses. That is, maybe you're not between the ages of nineteen and twenty-nine, like the men in the weightlifting study. And odds are you're not a long-distance runner, either. Sure, you might be saying to yourself, HMB works for *those* people. But it won't work for me.

Well, a study shows that HMB can work in people of just about *any* age . . . including seventy-year-olds.

Researchers at South Dakota State University gave either HMB or a placebo to fifteen men and sixteen women who had enrolled in a five-day-a-week program of resistance training. Their average age: seventy.

After eight weeks, those on the HMB gained three times more muscle and lost seven times more fat than the placebo group.

"HMB supplementation alters body composition during an 8-week exercise program in 70-year-old adults in a manner similar to its effect in young adults," wrote the researchers in the *Journal of Nutrition* in 2001. "This suggests that the underlying mechanism causing the stimulation of fat-free mass [muscle] gain is essentially independent of age."

Translation: young or old, HMB can work for you.

HMB: The Best Muscle-Building Supplement—Bar None

In 2002, Dr. Nissen and his colleagues at Iowa State University evaluated scientific studies done not only on HMB, but also on 250 other nutritional supplements touted as being able to boost the power of weightlifting to improve muscle size and strength. To be included in their review, the supplements had to be studied at least twice, with studies lasting three weeks or longer, and with resistance training occurring at least twice a week during the study. Only six supplements made the cut. They were:

- HMB

- creatine (an amino acid, and an energy source for muscle contraction)

- chromium (a trace mineral, discussed in Chapter 5 as a way to regulate the insulin system, reducing fat and adding muscle, but not as a way to improve the results of weight training)

- androstenedione (a precursor to the hormone testosterone, made famous—or infamous—by home run hitter Mark McGwire)

- dehydroepiandrosterone (DHEA, an adrenal hormone)

- protein supplements

Of these supplements, the researchers found that only two *really* improve muscle size and strength: HMB and creatine. At 3 grams a day, HMB improved muscle gains by an average of 0.28 percent a week more than placebo (creatine, 0.36 percent), and strength gain by 1.4 percent per week more than placebo (creatine, 1.1 percent).

"In summary," wrote Dr. Nissen in the February 2003 issue of the *Journal of Applied Physiology,* "of the 250 dietary products available, only HMB and creatine supplements have sufficient scientific evidence to conclude that lean body mass and strength gains accompanying resistance training are augmented."

HMB isn't HuMBug, that's for sure.

As for creatine: we're not talking about it in this book because *The Natural Fat-Loss Pharmacy* isn't primarily about supplements to help weightlifters and bodybuilders bulk up and get stronger. Yes, we want you to have more calorie-burning muscle and less fat. But more than that, we want you to stick with your exercise routine, by experiencing less soreness, fewer (or no) injuries, *and* real gains in firmness. Creatine can help you build muscle. But it doesn't necessarily *protect* muscle. HMB does.

It Doesn't Work If You Don't Exercise

HMB sounds great, no? So maybe you figure you'll take some HMB, build stronger, firmer muscles, and just *skip* the exercise. Sorry: HMB isn't a freebie. For it to work, you have to work out.

In a study of sedentary people, those who took HMB didn't show *any* change in muscle size or strength. But when the same people started a weightlifting program and took HMB, they had significant increases in muscle mass and strength, compared to a similar group of exercisers who took a placebo.

BEYOND EXERCISE

It's not only exercisers who need to preserve muscle. From aging to AIDS, many different diseases and developments can erode your muscles. HMB can slow down that loss.

Slowing Down (or Even Stopping!) Sarcopenia

To some degree, *everybody* over forty has "sarcopenia," or age-related muscle loss. It starts in your mid-thirties, with a yearly erosion of about

1 percent of your total muscle mass. It speeds up in your sixties. And by the time you're in your seventies, sarcopenia can be more of a disaster than a development. An elderly person with sarcopenia can become extremely frail and fall easily. What's more, as you lose muscle mass in your arms and legs, you also lose it in your diaphragm, making coughing much more difficult—and increasing the risk of death from pneumonia twentyfold, compared to older people with sarcopenia that's not as advanced.

HMB to the rescue.

Dr. Nissen gave HMB for one year to 120 men and women with an average age of seventy-five. Muscle loss was virtually *halted*. "This is the first time it's ever been demonstrated that you can prevent sarcopenia," he told us. "We think this is really big news." The study was reported at the 2006 Clinical Nutrition Week conference in Dallas, Texas.

Helping People with AIDS

Scientists studied forty-eight HIV-infected people who had lost at least 5 percent of their weight in the last three months. They divided them into two groups. For eight weeks, one group took a supplement consisting of HMB and the amino acids arginine and glutamine, and one group took a placebo. At the beginning and end of the study, the researchers measured body weight, as well as percentages of muscle and fat.

At the end of the study, those taking the HMB/amino combo had gained 6.6 pounds, as compared to 0.8 pounds for the placebo group. And 5.6 pounds of that weight gain was muscle.

Over the eight weeks, those taking HMB also developed stronger immune systems: they had more white blood cells and a decrease in their viral load of HIV.

"The data indicated that the HMB mixture can markedly alter the course of lean tissue loss in patients with AIDS-associated wasting," wrote the researchers, in the *Journal of Parenteral and Enteral Nutrition*.

Slowing Wasting in Advanced Cancer

As if advanced cancer weren't bad enough, it's often accompanied by *cancer cachexia*, in which patients lose a lot of weight, most of it in the form of muscle. HMB can help.

In a six-month study, published in the *American Journal of Surgery*, nine cancer patients received HMB (along with two other amino acids) or a placebo. After six months, those on the HMB/amino acid supplement had less weight loss and muscle wasting than those on the placebo. The positive results, say the researchers, "were similar to the positive changes in body composition observed in AIDS patients."

Protecting Your Heart

In studies on exercise, researchers often take a bevy of blood tests to see whether HMB is safe. Among those measurements are total cholesterol, LDL cholesterol (the "bad" cholesterol that lards arteries with plaque), and blood pressure.

In a review of nine such studies, Dr. Nissen found that people who took HMB had a greater drop in total cholesterol, LDL, and blood pressure than those taking a placebo.

Total cholesterol fell by 5.8 percent—particularly in people with total cholesterol of over 200 mg/dL or greater, the level that puts you at a higher risk for heart disease.

LDL cholesterol fell by 7.3 percent.

And systolic blood pressure (the top number) fell by 4.4 mm while diastolic (the bottom number) stayed the same.

"These effects," wrote Dr. Nissan in the *Journal of Nutrition* in 2000, "could result in a decrease in the risk of heart attack and stroke."

Not a bad boost for the heart-protecting power of exercise.

HOW TO TAKE HMB

Take the right dose. Three grams is the amount used in almost every study that shows positive results. But, says Dr. Nissen, people who weigh more than 200 pounds might benefit from 4 grams a day, and people who weigh 120 pounds or less could use 1 or 1.5 grams. If you're an older person trying to prevent sarcopenia, Dr. Nissen recommends 2 grams a day.

Once a day is fine. When should you take HMB? "We've studied this question extensively and our answer is—it doesn't seem to make much of a difference," says Dr. Nissen. "Before exercise, after exercise, with meals, between meals—there's no real evidence to show that any of that makes any difference in the effectiveness of HMB."

Instead, says Dr. Nissen, take the supplement in a way that guarantees you're going to take it day after day, year after year. "And that's probably not taking three capsules, three times a day," he says. "If you're an everyday exerciser or an older person who is taking HMB to preserve muscle, once a day is fine. If you're a bodybuilder or endurance athlete, take it twice a day, in equally spaced doses."

Use HMB by itself, not in a combination product. There are many brands of HMB on the market. Pick a supplement with *only* HMB, for proven results. "Stick with the plainest and simplest product out there," says Dr. Nissen. "Don't waste your money on products with multiple ingredients."

Buy a brand you trust. "We've tested many imported products in our lab and many have been of questionable purity," says Dr. Nissen. Stick with a brand you know and trust. In his studies, Dr. Nissen has used the HMB manufactured by EAS bodybuilding and nutrition supplements.

HMB IS SAFE

Scientists have looked closely and carefully at the safety of HMB—and declared it to be *very* safe.

Once again, Dr. Nissen has conducted the best research on the topic. He says many studies in which HMB was fed to a wide variety of animals showed no adverse effects on health—in fact, the animals typically got healthier. And a couple of studies on humans indicate HMB is safe. But to make sure, he looked at safety data in nine studies on people, where at least 3 grams of HMB were given per day, for three to eight weeks.

Seven of the studies were conducted by Dr. Nissen and his colleagues at Iowa State University, one was conducted at Wichita State University in Kansas, and one at Ball State University in Indiana. The studies looked at men and women, at the young and old, and at exercisers and non-exercisers.

The scientists measured organ and tissue function (as evaluated by blood tests); any emotional changes (what's the use of taking a supplement that helps your muscles but messes with your head?); and general health, through a questionnaire that asked HMB takers to answer thirty-two health-related queries.

Dr. Nissen's conclusion: "No untoward effects of HMB were indicated."

In fact, people who took HMB reported a *decrease* in a category of emotional health called "unactivated unpleasant affect," which is described as feeling dull, tired, drowsy, sluggish, bored, and droopy. (Sounds like six of the seven dwarves, on a very bad day.)

The data from these nine experiments, wrote Dr. Nissen, in the *Journal of Nutrition*, "suggest that the popular use of supplemental HMB at 3 grams a day as an ergogenic [nutritional] aid for exercise is well tolerated and safe in humans."

Relax and take HMB. On second thought, *don't* relax. Exercise and take HMB. Your muscles will thank you.

BCAA: THE THREE AMINOS

We've just finished talking about HMB, a metabolite of leucine, an essential amino acid. (There are twenty amino acids, the molecular components of protein. Nine are *essential*, meaning it's essential to get them from the diet, because the body doesn't make them.)

Now, we'll look at a supplement that's a mixture of leucine and two other essential amino acids, isoleucine and valine. These are the *branched-chain amino acids* (BCAA), a term describing their chemical architecture. They comprise 35 percent of the amino acids in muscle tissue. And, as you might have guessed, what makes them particularly important players in the fate of your waistline is the way they affect your muscles.

Studies show that BCAA (like HMB) can *prevent* muscle breakdown and *trigger* muscle building. That means supplying your muscles with extra BCAA can (again, like HMB) help prevent exercise-related muscle damage: soreness after exercise, and the likelihood of a sprain, strain, or other injury. They can also help your body build more calorie-burning muscle. Let's take a closer look.

Down by the DNA

Although nobody knows exactly how BCAA works to protect and build muscle, there are a few theories.

Muscle-building messages. BCAA may activate RNA—the molecules that carry messages from the DNA in the cell's nucleus to the rest of the cell, passing on orders to create more protein.

Muscle-protecting fuel. Most essential amino acids are burned in the liver for fuel. But BCAA can be burned right in the muscle—and is, particularly during exercise. When muscles burn BCAA for fuel, they seem to get added protection from protein breakdown.

Muscle-repairing signals. BCAA may also work by allowing the cell to receive signals that tell it to repair.

In a study conducted by researchers at the University College of Physical Education and Sports, in Stockholm, Sweden, researchers gave BCAA to seven men and then had them perform a session of resistance training on their quadriceps, the muscles of the front of the thigh. Before, during, and after the exercise, the men got a drink containing either BCAA or a placebo.

In the hours after the exercise, the researchers took four measurements of *protein kinase*, enzymes that activate other proteins by adding the mineral phosphate to the mix. This process is called *phosphorylation*, and it's crucial to normal cellular function (including muscle cells). The researchers noted that, in both the BCAA and the placebo groups, resistance exercise led to a "robust increase" in the phosphorylation of three of their markers. But the BCAA group had *much* larger increases in phosphorylation during the *recovery* period.

This increase is a sure sign, they say, of BCAA's effect on *signal transduction*: the ability of the muscle cells to receive signals from outside the cell—in this case, the signal to *repair*.

But however BCAA does it, the fact that it protects and builds muscles is obvious—from the results of lots of scientific studies.

Less Muscle Damage

Earlier in the chapter, we told you about studies on athletes and HMB, with scientists measuring levels of three chemicals produced when protein breaks down: CK, LDH, and 3-MH. In a similar study on BCAA, researchers at the Center for Human Movement at the University of Tasmania in Australia tested sixteen men, giving one group BCAA and the other a placebo. After seven days, both groups got an exercise test—they cycled two hours on a stationary bicycle. Then CK and LDH were measured.

In both groups, CK and LDH were much higher after exercising, as would be expected. But those who took BCAA had significantly lower levels of LDH from two hours to five days after the endurance exercise, and significantly lower CK levels from four hours to five days after the exercise.

"BCAA supplementation may reduce the muscle damage associated with endurance exercise," wrote the scientists in the *Journal of Sports Medicine and Physical Fitness* in 2004.

Get a Grip—With BCAA

Italian researchers gave BCAA or a placebo to ten healthy men for thirty days. Before they started taking BCAA, the men were measured for the total area of muscle on their arms, the strength of their grip, and the amount of oxygen they consumed during the grip test. (In other words, did performing the grip exercise make them breathe more heavily?) The same measurements were taken after thirty days.

Stronger. The BCAA group had a significant increase in their grip strength compared to the placebo group.

Fitter. The men taking the grip test who didn't get BCAA needed a lot more oxygen than the men taking BCAA.

"BCAA supplementation improved the physical fitness of untrained healthy subjects, as demonstrated by the lack of O_2 uptake increase during a sustained hand grip test," the researchers wrote in *Diabetes, Nutrition and Metabolism* in 2003.

Beat the Heat

Scientists in the Department of Exercise Science at Rutgers University wanted to see if BCAA would help endurance exercisers cope with heat. They had thirteen people (seven men and six women) cycle to exhaustion (at a moderate pace) in 94 degrees Fahrenheit. Every thirty minutes during the exercise, they gave them a drink with either BCAA or a placebo.

Those getting BCAA cycled for 153 minutes; those getting the placebo, 137.

"These results indicate BCAA supplementation prolongs moderate exercise performance in the heat," they wrote in *Medicine and Science in Sports and Exercise.*

A Mountain of Muscle

Italian researchers from the University of Verona gave either BCAA or a placebo to sixteen people who trekked for twenty-one days at altitudes ranging from ten thousand to eleven thousand feet—a situation in which muscle can be lost because of the intense exercise and lower levels of tissue-nourishing oxygen. There were noticeable differences in the two groups after the twenty-one-day hike was finished.

Predictably, body fat decreased in both groups. But overall muscle increased by 1.5 percent in the BCAA group, while there was little change in the placebo group. Arm muscle increased in the BCAA group, while it decreased by 6.8 percent in the placebo group. And the BCAA group had 5 percent more strength in their legs than the placebo group.

Feeling Less Fatigued During Endurance Exercise

In a study by Swedish scientists, endurance-trained cyclists received either BCAA or a placebo during exercise. During the exercise, the cyclists rated their "perceived exertion" (how hard they felt they were exercising) and their mental fatigue. Those getting BCAA had a 7 percent lower level of perceived exertion and a 15 percent lower level of mental fatigue.

Explanation: Exercise scientists say there are two kinds of fatigue: *peripheral fatigue*, in the muscles themselves; and *central fatigue*, where you just *feel* a lot more fatigued. They know what causes peripheral fatigue: blood sugar delivery to muscles is low and lactate (an acid produced in muscles during exercise) is high. But nobody really understands the causes of central fatigue. One theory from European scientists, supported by research, suggests that low levels of BCAA are the cause of central fatigue. Here's how it might happen:

1. Increases in the brain chemical serotonin put the body in a lower gear, creating feelings of sleepiness or fatigue.

2. When the amino acid tryptophan enters the brain, it creates more serotonin—and more tryptophan enters the brain during exercise.

3. To get into the brain, tryptophan must cross the *blood–brain barrier*.

SHOULD YOU TAKE HMB OR BCAA?

Both supplements sound good, and both seem to do pretty much the same thing: protect and build muscle. So how do you decide between the two?

"I'm not sure that there's an answer to that question," says Sid Stohs, PhD, of the School of Pharmacy and Health Professions, Creighton University Medical Center, and a scientist who has studied both supplements. "A person can read about HMB and BCAA, but which you decide to take really comes down to what works for you. My recommendation: decide to take one and see whether or not you get results. If you do, continue to take that supplement. If you don't, try the other one and proceed from there. I think the reality of choosing HMB or BCAA is really a matter of personal experimentation."

Steve Nissen, PhD, a professor at Iowa State University who has conducted much of the research on HMB, has a slightly different opinion: he favors HMB.

"I've spent my life studying branched-chain amino acids," he told us. "I know they can improve protein synthesis. But when you really come down to what the effect is in *people* in terms of muscle protection and gain, I think there is far more consistent, reliable scientific data for HMB than for BCAA."

4. If there are competing amino acids like BCAA trying to get across the *carrier system* that allows nutrients to cross the barrier, then less tryptophan gets to the brain.

More BCAA = less tryptophan in the brain during exercise = less serotonin = less central fatigue.

Stronger Immune Systems in Endurance Exercisers

It's a well-known fact among exercise scientists that intense endurance exercise wears out the immune system, probably by lowering blood levels of the amino acid glutamine. Scientists in Brazil gave either BCAA or a placebo to twelve elite male triathletes who participated in the 1997 and 1998 São Paolo International Triathlons. (This triathlon involved a swim of 1.5 kilometers, or 0.93 miles; a bike ride of 40 kilometers, or 24.8 miles; and a run of 10 kilometers, or 6.2 miles.)

After the triathlon, the athletes getting the placebo had lower levels of glutamine; the athletes getting BCAA didn't. The placebo group also had a 22 percent decrease in infection-fighting white bloods cells called *lymphocytes*; the BCAA group didn't. And the BCAA group reported 33 percent fewer symptoms of infection than the placebo group.

The study was published in the July 2000 issue of *Medicine and Science in Sports and Exercise.*

BCAA and Other Health Problems

BCAA doesn't just affect muscle. It plays a key role in *many* different processes in the body—and can often affect them for the better.

Liver disease. Although it's controversial, many liver specialists think that BCAA can help with symptoms of liver disease (cirrhosis), a common problem among alcoholics and those with hepatitis C. Why BCAA for liver disease?

People with liver disease tend to metabolize even more protein than natural. Also, there's a 65 to 90 percent incidence of protein malnutrition in those with cirrhosis. BCAA may help preserve or restore muscle in people with liver disease.

Those with liver disease can also have brain and nervous system damage (hepatic encephalopathy) and BCAA can improve these symptoms. (We'll tell you more about BCAA and the brain in a moment.)

And BCAA may even delay liver failure and death in patients with cirrhosis.

In a study conducted by Italian researchers and published in the June 2003 issue of *Gastroenterology*, 174 patients with advanced cirrhosis were given either BCAA supplements or non-BCAA nutritional supplementation. Those on BCAA had significantly fewer cases of liver failure or death.

They also had a lower rate of hospital admissions, better appetite, and a higher "quality of life."

Neurological and emotional problems. BCAA affects neurotransmitters, the chemicals that help send messages from brain cell to brain cell—which means BCAA may improve diseases of the brain and nervous system.

Mania. British doctors at the University of Oxford gave twenty-five manic-depressive patients a drink containing either BCAA or a placebo for seven days. BCAA lowered symptoms of mania "acutely" during the first six hours after the drink and provided a "persistent advantage" over the week, said the researchers, in the *British Journal of Psychiatry* in March 2003.

Tardive dyskinesia. People who take *neuroleptic drugs* daily for long-term psychiatric and neurological problems can end up with a grotesque side effect—involuntary, repetitive facial movements like grimacing or lip smacking, and rapid movements of the arms, legs, or fingers.

Researchers at the Division of Movement Disorders and Molecular Psychiatry at the Nathan S. Kline Institute for Psychiatric Research in New York gave BCAA or a placebo for three weeks to thirty-six patients with tardive dyskinesia. Symptoms were reduced within one week.

"Branched-chain amino acids constitute a novel, safe treatment for tardive dyskinesia, with a strong potential for providing significant improvement in the diseased physiognomy of the afflicted person," wrote the researchers, in the June 2003 issue of the *American Journal of Psychiatry*.

Spinocerebellar degeneration (SCD). This is a general term for nervous system degeneration caused by hereditary diseases, stroke, multiple sclerosis, or other problems. It results in *ataxia,* or balance and coordination problems.

Japanese doctors gave BCAA or a placebo for four weeks to sixteen people with SCD. The symptoms improved significantly in the BCAA group, with no change in the placebo group.

In the March 2002 issue of the *Journal of Neurological Sciences,* the doctors reported that "treatment with BCAA may be effective" in patients with SCD.

Is It Safe?

BCAA is part of protein—part of *food*. It's *essential*—you can't live without it. And because the body needs it, BCAA is very unlikely to do you any harm, even in the large doses found in supplements. Toxicity studies on animals—in which huge doses are given to produce negative results—showed no negative effects, except at massive doses. There has never been a single report about health problems from taking a BCAA supplement.

"There is very little evidence in [animals] or humans that BCAAs are toxic except at very high doses," wrote scientists from Wake Forest University School of Medicine, in a paper on safe intakes of BCAA.

How Much Should You Take?

In most of the studies reported in this chapter, researchers used 5 grams or more per day. Most BCAA products offer 1-gram capsules, with a mixture of the three amino acids. Pick a brand you trust and follow the dosage recommendations on the label.

PART VII

Thermogenics

11

Calorie-Burning Metabolism Boosters—For Now, Cross Them Off Your Fat-Loss Shopping List

- Ephedra, Citrus Aurantium, Caffeine

Why are we telling you about a type of weight-loss supplement that we *don't* think you should take? Because they're widely available, and it's important for you to know why they're not a good choice at this time.

WHAT IS THERMOGENESIS?

The supplements discussed in this chapter are *thermogenics*. They work by triggering *thermogenesis*.

Thermogenesis is your body's way of saying, "Let there be heat!" It's what happens when metabolism—your body's calorie-burning mechanism—speeds up.

Scientifically speaking, there are three widely recognized, nondrug ways to increase thermogenesis:

- TEF (thermogenic effect of food): the extra calories you burn when the body digests and absorbs what you just ate.

- AT (activity thermogenesis): the extra calories you burn when you engage in an exercise like walking, jogging, or biking.

- NEAT (non-exercise activity thermogenesis): the extra calories you burn when you're strolling in the mall or combing your hair or doing just about anything except sleeping or resting (a baseline condition called *resting metabolic rate*, or RMR).

If you increase thermogenesis, you increase calorie burning. If you burn more calories than you take in, you lose weight.

Unfortunately, it's not always that simple, says Arne Astrup, MD, the head of the Department of Human Nutrition at RVA University in Copenhagen, Denmark, and one of the world's leading experts on using thermogenics to lose weight.

Yes, he says, the best way to take off (and keep off) the pounds is to control calorie intake and exercise regularly.

But some people may find that harder than others because of what scientists call their *phenotype*: a combination of genes and learned habits (with the emphasis on the genes) produces a lower-than-average resting metabolic rate, with 5 to 8 percent fewer calories burned per day.

And even if your RMR is normal and you manage to lose weight, a second factor can kick in. After you lose weight, your resting metabolic rate tends to fall by 3 to 5 percent—*permanently*. That makes it quite hard to maintain weight loss, because you have to eat *less* to stay at the *same* weight.

What can you do if you're in one of these categories that Dr. Astrup describes? You can't seem to make the pounds budge. Or you've lost weight and gained it back. Or you don't want to starve yourself for the rest of your life dealing with either of those two issues. Well, he says, you can take a *thermogenic*.

Thermogenics have a big, scientific-sounding name, but they're everywhere in our daily diet. Coffee (or any substance containing caffeine) is a thermogenic. Nicotine is a thermogenic. Thermogenics stimulate your nervous system. They tighten muscles, speed your heart, and boost your blood pressure. You're in fifth gear, and the body burns more fuel—more calories and more fat—to keep you there.

In summary: thermogenics speed up your nervous system, requiring your body to burn more calories.

Maybe you're thinking, "I'll take one of those!"

Well, millions of Americans did take one: the thermogenic *ephedra*. Many lost weight. But at what cost to health?

EPHEDRA: AN HERB TO DIE FOR

Let's start at the end (or at least one of the last chapters) of the ephedra story.

On April 12, 2004, the government's Food and Drug Agency (FDA) banned supplements containing the herb.

Ephedrine, the synthetic form of ephedra, had long been available as an ingredient in OTC drugs for asthma, nasal congestion, and minor eye irritation and was regulated by the FDA. But in the 1990s, natural ephedrine, from the Chinese herb *ma huang*, began appearing in OTC products that promised to trim the body, boost energy, or improve athletic performance. Because it was a supplement, natural ephedrine wasn't regulated by the FDA. And it became hugely popular, with 2 to 3 billion doses of the pill taken yearly. How exactly does ephedra work to promote weight loss?

Ephedrine is a *beta agonist*. (An *agonist* is the opposite of an *antagonist*: it stimulates rather than opposes.) Beta agonists stimulate the beta receptors of the sympathetic nervous system. This is the part of the nervous system that controls the *fight-or-flight response*—the body's emergency switch for instant action. Perceive a threat—real or imagined—and the heart beats faster, breathing becomes more rapid, blood pressure rises, and digestion slows. (Emergencies are no time for your next meal.) You're raring to go—to battle or skedaddle.

As a class of drugs, beta agonists are labeled *sympathmimetics* because they mimic the action of the sympathetic nervous system. And ephedrine is a particularly effective sympathmimetic. It increases body temperature, boosting calorie burning. It speeds up fat burning. It mutes appetite. It energizes. Unfortunately, as we said, it also can raise heart rate, blood pressure . . . and safety issues.

Hurting the Heart

Researchers at the University of California, San Francisco (UCSF) and the California Poison Control System reviewed 140 cases of "adverse events" associated with ephedra that were reported to the FDA from June 1997 to March 1999. They concluded that forty-three cases were "definitely or probably" related to ephedra and another forty-four were "possibly" related.

They tallied seventeen cases of high blood pressure, thirteen of rapid or irregular heartbeat, ten strokes, and seven seizures.

There were ten deaths, and thirteen people were permanently disabled.

There was the case of the healthy thirty-five-year-old woman who began taking ephedra for weight loss. One week later, she collapsed during an aerobics class—with a heart attack and a ruptured blood vessel in her brain.

There was the case of a healthy thirty-nine-year-old man who downed an ephedra-rich drink a few minutes after his three-mile run—and started experiencing numbness in his right arm and leg. He'd had a mild stroke.

"Because of the severity of the adverse events that we reviewed, and, in particular, the occurrence of events that caused permanent disability or death, we conclude that dietary supplements that contain ephedra . . . pose a serious health risk to some users," wrote the researchers in the *New England Journal of Medicine* in 2000.

Ephedra Psychosis

Ephedra, another study showed, isn't just risky for the body. It can also drive you mad.

Researchers at RAND, a nonprofit research institute in California, reviewed all the adverse events associated with ephedra, focusing on psychiatric problems.

They reported fifty-seven cases of "psychosis, severe depression, mania or agitation, hallucinations, sleep disturbances, and suicidal ideation [thoughts about committing suicide]" after people had taken ephedra. (Most of these people had preexisting psychiatric problems and were taking other mood-altering drugs.) In ten of these cases, people hurt themselves; in five, they hurt somebody else.

"Clinicians should be aware that serious psychiatric symptoms could be associated with ephedra use," wrote the researchers in the *American Journal of Psychiatry*.

Sales: 1 Percent; Side Effects: 64 Percent

A study by researchers at the Osher Center for Integrative Medicine at UCSF looked at all the adverse events from herbal products in the U.S.— and concluded that ephedra was responsible for 64 percent of them, even though ephedra products represented less than 1 percent of sales.

"Ephedra use is associated with a greatly increased risk for adverse reactions compared with other herbs, and its use should be restricted," wrote the authors, in the March 2003 issue of the *Annals of Internal Medicine*.

Not Everybody Hates Ephedra

The millions of people who took ephedra weren't doing so because they were thrill seekers who wanted to flirt with cardiac disaster. They wanted to lose weight. And many did.

Numerous scientific studies show that ephedra can help people shed pounds and fat, particularly when it's combined with caffeine. (We'll talk about caffeine's thermogenic-assisting power in a minute.)

In one of the best of these studies, researchers from the New York Obesity Research Center at Columbia University looked at 167 healthy but overweight men and women. They divided them into two groups: one got an ephedra/caffeine mixture (90 milligrams (mg) a day of ephedra and 192 mg of caffeine) and the other a placebo. After six months, the ephedra/caffeine group had lost 11.7 pounds, while the placebo group had lost 5.7. The ephedra/caffeine group also lost 50 percent more fat than the placebo group.

But was ephedra safe? Yes. The ephedra/caffeine group had, on average, a very small increase in heart rate (four beats per minute) and blood pressure (three to five points). There were no heart palpitations or irregular heartbeats.

"In this 6-month placebo-controlled trial, herbal ephedra/caffeine promoted body weight and body fat reduction . . . without significant adverse events," wrote the researchers in the May 2002 issue of the *International Journal of Obesity*.

Two years earlier, in 2000, an independent scientific research firm issued the Cantox Report, which looked at the "strong scientific findings" on ephedrine and ephedra from dozens of studies conducted by researchers from all over the world between 1974 and 2000. They concluded that ephedra was safe and effective when used in a split dosage: three pills per day, with no pill exceeding 30 mg.

They concluded that "90 mg of ephedrine alkaloids in ephedra per day for a generally healthy population . . . is unlikely to pose a risk of adverse health effects."

We present these pro-ephedra findings because we don't want to demonize the herb. It can work. In fact, many physicians (including Dr. Preuss) think that ephedra is the most effective natural weight-loss supplement. The question, of course, is whether the negative effects are excessive. But taken at the suggested dose, and with the proper medical supervision and precautions (people with high blood pressure and other cardiovascular risk factors should avoid ephedra), the risk–benefit ratio is acceptable— especially in light of the rising rates of obesity.

Nevertheless, with so many other weight-loss aids available, and because of the legal implications for doctors who prescribe the herb, Dr. Preuss says ephedra is *not* a supplement for everyday use.

EPHEDRA ALKALOIDS: DON'T TAKE THEM LIGHTLY

Ephedra is the name of a species of Asian plants, which includes the Chinese herb *ma huang*. All varieties of ephedra contain *alkaloids*, a class of compounds produced by plants—and sometimes craved by humans. (Nicotine and caffeine are alkaloids, for example.)

There's *ephedrine*, the most active ingredient, comprising anywhere from 40 to 90 percent of the alkaloids in ephedra.

There's *pseudoephedrine*, which is used in nasal decongestants and cold remedies—and also in the illegal manufacture of methamphetamine. (In 2006, the Senate and House passed a bill requiring that OTC products with pseudoephedrine be kept behind the pharmacy counter or in a locked cabinet and be sold only to customers with IDs who sign a logbook, with no customer allowed to buy more than 9 grams per month.)

And there's *phenylpropanolamine*, also found in OTC cough-and-cold products, decongestants, and weight-loss pills—and another denizen of meth labs. In 2000, the FDA called for manufacturers to voluntarily discontinue marketing products with phenylpropanolamine after a Yale study suggested that users of products containing the ingredient were at a higher risk of stroke than nonusers.

As you can see, ephedra alkaloids are tough customers. Don't take them lightly.

The Resurrection of Ephedra

Maybe you thought ephedra was *banned*. As in banished, exiled, forbidden, vanished, gone. But just when you thought it was safe to go back to the health food store again . . . ephedra has returned.

A Utah-based supplement company sued the FDA over the ban on ephedra. In April 2005, a federal district court judge in Utah ruled that smaller dosages of ephedra posed no threat to public health, and that the company could market ephedra in dosages of 10 mg or less. Ephedra is back on the market. But that's not keeping the FDA from trying to stop it.

In 2006, the agency seized two hundred cases of finished product (with supplements containing more than 10 mg), two hundred boxes of bulk tablets, and nine 25-kilo drums of raw material with ephedrine.

"We will continue to do all we can to protect the public health against these dietary supplements that have been found to cause serious illness and injury," said the acting FDA commissioner.

Stay tuned for Round 3.

CITRUS AURANTIUM: ORANGE ALERT

In 2004, with ephedra more or less out of the picture, many supplement companies replaced it with another thermogenic: *citrus aurantium*.

Citrus aurantium is the botanical name for a citrus fruit that also goes by Bitter Orange, Seville Orange, and China Orange. Its homeland is Asia (it's called *Zhi shi* in Chinese, *Kijitsu* in Japanese, and *Chisil* in Korean), where it has a long history of use as an herb for digestive disorders. The small, fifteen-foot orange tree produces oranges with a skin a bit rougher and darker than the oranges in supermarkets in America.

And these oranges are unique in another way: they contain *synephrine*, a sympathmimetic similar to ephedrine.

Unlike ephedrine, however, synephrine may work by targeting *beta 3* receptors (which boost calorie and fat burning) and bypass *beta 1* and *beta 2* receptors (which speed up heart rate and raise blood pressure).

A Study or Two

A few small studies show that citrus aurantium may help people lose weight.

In a study published in *Current Therapeutic Research*, twenty-three overweight men and women were put on a diet and exercise program for six weeks. One group got a supplement containing 975 mg of citrus aurantium and 528 mg of caffeine; one group got a placebo; one group got nothing.

On average, the supplement group lost 7 pounds of body fat and 3 pounds of weight. Those in the other groups didn't lose much weight at all. And the people taking the supplement suffered no side effects: no increase in blood pressure or heart rate; no changes in electrocardiogram readings; no odd signs in blood chemistry or urinalysis.

But a single positive study doesn't necessarily mean citrus aurantium is effective—or safe.

Researchers in the School of Pharmacy at UCSF gave fifteen young, healthy men and women a single dose of 900 mg of bitter orange or a placebo and then measured blood pressure and heart rate every hour for the next six hours.

Those who took bitter orange had an average increase of 7.3 points in systolic blood pressure, 2.6 points in diastolic blood pressure, and 4.2 beats per minute in heart rate.

In another study at UCSF, people received weight-loss supplements containing either citrus aurantium or a placebo for a week. Once again, systolic and diastolic blood pressure went up (9.6 and 9.1 points), as did heart rate (16.7 beats per minute with one product; 11.4 beats per minute with another).

"Ephedra-free weight loss supplements have significant cardiovascular stimulant actions, similar to ephedra," wrote the UCSF researchers in the September 2005 issue of the *American Journal of Medicine*.

Other headlines in scientific journals have warned doctors and scientists about citrus aurantium. For example . . .

- "Adverse reaction to an adrenergic herbal extract (Citrus aurantium)," in *Phytomedicine*

- "Potential for toxicity with use of bitter orange extract and guarana for weight loss," in the *Annals of Pharmacotherapy*

- "Products containing bitter orange or synephrine: suspected cardiovascular adverse reactions," in the *Canadian Medical Association Journal*

And a couple of really scary ones . . .

- "Possible association of acute lateral-wall myocardial infarction [heart attack] and bitter orange supplement," in *Annals of Pharmacotherapy*

- "Ischemic stroke associated with use of an ephedra-free dietary supplement containing synephrine," in *Mayo Clinic Proceedings*

In the first case, a fifty-five-year-old woman went to an emergency room with the classic symptoms of a heart attack: dull, aching shoulder and chest pain. It turned out that she was having one—and that for the past year she had been taking a daily weight-loss supplement with 300 mg of bitter orange.

"The use of C. aurantium-containing supplements may present as a risk for cardiovascular toxicity," wrote the researchers, in the *Annals of Pharmacotherapy*.

In the second case, a thirty-eight-year-old man who had been taking one or two capsules a day of an ephedra-free product with synephrine for a week showed up at a hospital with a slightly impaired walk and severe problems with memory and concentration. He had no history of circulatory problems and wasn't taking any other medication. A CAT scan and an MRI showed that he'd had a small stroke. After a few days, his symptoms cleared up.

"Synephrine . . . may be associated with ischemic stroke," wrote the researchers in *Mayo Clinic Proceedings*. "Consumers and clinicians need to be informed about the potential risks of ephedra-free products."

At this point, it's probably no surprise to be told that Dr. Preuss does *not* recommend citrus aurantium for weight loss. Yes, it *might* be a substitute for ephedra, but much more research would have to be conducted to prove that fact. And its safety is still not proven. For now, if you see "bitter orange" (or "citrus aurantium" or "synephrine") on the label of a weight-loss product, consider it an orange alert. (But don't worry about eating Seville oranges: citrus aurantium is derived from the *skin* of the orange.)

CAFFEINE: STICK WITH SMALL DOSES

If you're anything like the average American, you already know the pleasurable power of caffeine, found in coffee, cola, and energy drinks. Caf-

THE MANY FACES OF CAFFEINE

Many weight-loss products on the marketplace are basically caffeine pills. But you may not even *see* caffeine on the label. Instead, you'll see other ingredients that are rich in caffeine or caffeine-like substances. They might include:

Kola nut. Once upon a time, kola was the cola in cola drinks—a high-caffeine nut, native to West Africa and Indonesia. (Today, the cola flavor is more likely to be artificial.)

Guarana. Guarana is a plant from Brazil and Venezuela with seeds rich in guaranine, a chemical very similar to caffeine.

Yerba maté. This South American herb—a species of holly—is dried, chopped, and powdered to create a tea or herbal extract rich in xanthines, a substance similar to caffeine.

feine works most of its wake-up wonders by stimulating the sympathetic nervous system, which means it also boosts thermogenesis—and burns calories and fat.

Eighty more calories a day. In a study reported in the *American Journal of Clinical Nutrition*, people who had just lost weight took 100 mg of caffeine every two hours while awake. (There are about 100 mg of caffeine in an 8-ounce cup of brewed coffee.) They burned 80 calories more a day than other people who had just lost weight who didn't take caffeine supplements.

"Caffeine at commonly consumed doses can have a significant effect on energy balance [calories burned]," and may be useful "in the treatment of obesity," the researchers concluded.

Caffeine is also the perfect sidekick to ephedra and other thermogenics, boosting their effectiveness. And, in fact, in Chapter 1, on green tea extract, Dr. Preuss recommends as maximally effective a supplement containing EGCG *and* 150 mg of caffeine. But how about caffeine on its own as a way to lose weight? Not a good idea, says Dr. Preuss.

Large amounts of caffeine can make you anxious, cause insomnia, and stress your circulatory system. And the problem with most weight-loss supplements containing caffeine is that *you don't know how much caffeine is in them.* They can include not only caffeine, but also caffeine-containing herbs like kola nut, yerba maté, and guarana. Essentially, you're trying to lose weight by taking a high-dose caffeine pill. And high-dose caffeine pills aren't good for you.

Caffeine pills make stress worse. In a study conducted by researchers in the Department of Psychiatry and Behavioral Sciences at Duke University Medical Center, coffee drinkers were given either a 500 mg caffeine pill or a placebo for three days. Those taking the pill had higher heart rates and blood pressure, higher urinary levels of *catecholamines* and *cortisol,* stress hormones generated by the adrenal glands—and "higher levels of self-reported stress" during the activities of the day.

A caffeine pill isn't a safe, healthy way to help yourself lose weight. Have a cup or two of coffee instead!

PART VIII

The Natural Fat-Loss
Prescription

12

The Natural Fat-Loss Pharmacy Supplement Program
Designing the Approach That's Right for You

You've read about the fat busters EGCG, CLA, HCA, and MCT. About the insulin regulator chromium. About carbohydrate inhibitors that block the digestion of starch and sugar. About filling fiber and calming 5-HTP. About the muscle builders HMB and BCAA. You've read about them . . . you're convinced they can help you safely lose weight, shed fat, firm up, or maintain weight . . . and you want to turn that conviction into results. But there are still a few questions . . .

Which one should you take? Should you take *more* than one? How do you design a weight-loss supplement program that's right for *you*? This chapter will help you answer those very questions.

PARTNER WITH A PROFESSIONAL

It's important to remember that weight loss isn't just about designing a *supplement* program. The key to weight loss, fat loss, muscle gain, or weight maintenance is a calorie-smart diet and regular exercise. The supplements discussed in *The Natural Fat-Loss Pharmacy* are *aids* to such a program—and never a substitute for it.

And a program that addresses nutrition, exercise, and supplements is best designed and monitored not on your own, but in close consultation with a health professional, like a doctor or nutritionist. That professional can help you decide which supplements to use, taking into account factors like . . .

Your preferences, goals, and health problems. Maybe you've experimented with a fiber supplement and just didn't like it. Maybe your goal is maintaining your weight, not losing more pounds. Maybe your blood sugar is high. Maybe you want to reduce the impact of a fatty diet. How does each supplement match *your* life—and which are the best match?

What works for you. People are individuals. Not each supplement will work for everyone. Under the supervision of a health professional, you can experiment, finding the supplement that works best for you. And if it doesn't work, you can switch.

The optimum combinations. Supplements don't have to be taken singly—you can combine them for maximum effect.

Two Experts in Weight-Loss Supplementation

Equipped with the information and ideas in this book, sit down and work with a doctor, nutritionist, or other health professional to create a personalized supplement plan.

And to help you work with a professional, we talked with two of the best: doctors who have treated thousands of patients for weight loss, recommending one or more of the supplements discussed in this book:

Leigh Erin Connealy, MD, MPH, is the medical director of the South Coast Medical Center for New Medicine, in Tustin, California (www.

scmedicalcenter.com). Dr. Connealy works with a staff of two other doctors, two nurse practitioners, a certified nutritionist, two licensed acupuncturists, a specialist in energy medicine, and a certified aromatherapist. "We focus on therapies other than drugs or surgery—natural therapies that support the body's healing mechanisms and innate defenses," says Dr. Connealy.

Tammy L. Born, DO, is the director of the Born Preventive Health Care Clinics in Grand Rapids, Michigan, and Goshen, Indiana (www.bornclinic. com). The Michigan clinic is staffed by five other physicians, including a naturopathic physician, and a certified acupuncturist. "We specialize in finding the *cause* of a health problem, not just treating the effects," says Dr. Born.

The Doctor–Patient Team

Both Drs. Connealy and Born think that a good doctor–patient relationship is the key to determining the weight-loss supplements that are right for you—and to making sure that you take them regularly, and that they're working.

"If you're trying to lose weight, you need a health professional to be in touch with regularly," says Dr. Connealy. "The more accountable you are to a doctor or other health professional—accountable about your diet, exercise, and supplements—the more likely it is you're going to stick with your program and be successful in reaching your weight-loss goals."

"Go to a physician who can help keep you accountable," agrees Dr. Born. "Form a team with your doctor—set goals, write them down, and achieve them. That's the approach that works."

Profiles in Supplementation

In the rest of the chapter, we'll review the supplements one by one, listing the factors that might indicate a supplement is right for you.

We'll also present a patient profile for every supplement—real-life stories of weight-loss patients seen by Dr. Connealy, and the supplements she recommended (both for weight loss *and* general health).

EGCG (GREEN TEA EXTRACT)

"Green tea is good for almost everyone," says Dr. Connealy. "I drink green tea. I have my kids drink green tea. I serve green tea in the waiting room."

"Green tea is such a great antioxidant," agrees Dr. Born. "And it also has powerful anti-inflammatory effects, so we can use green tea extract to help prevent or treat every disease that involves inflammation, from arthritis to Alzheimer's to cancer to diabetes to heart disease."

For weight loss, Dr. Born recommends EGCG particularly for people who feel tired all the time. She says, "I also give it to overweight people who complain of 'brain fog,' and who have arthritis or a family history of the disease."

Consider taking EGCG if . . .

- You want to prevent weight gain.

- You want to maintain weight loss.

- You want a safe alternative to ephedra.

- You want to boost the power of your workout to burn fat.

- You feel tired all the time.

- You have arthritis, or another disease involving inflammation.

- You want better health, including possible protection against aging, high blood fats, various cancers, and immune problems.

KIM: She wants to look great for *herself*
EGCG, chromium, 5-HTP, chitosan

Dr. Connealy: Kim is a stay-at-home mom with three teenage girls and a six-year-old son with autism. Every day she feels ill prepared, and that she is somehow responsible for her son's autism. She cries frequently. And she likes to sneak food when no one is around, to relieve stress and for the comfort it provides.

Her maternal aunt has diabetes and recently lost her left leg due to complications of diabetes. Her father died three years ago at fifty-nine from a massive stroke. Her mother lives in another state and only calls to criticize her, which is very upsetting and depressing to Kim.

Kim married Kevin, her first love, right after high school, and they moved to California. They are both thirty-six years old. Kevin deals with his son's autism by working late and often being out of town.

In marriage counseling, Kevin recently admitted to having an affair. He says he's no longer attracted to Kim, and blames her for all the stress in their poorly kept home.

Kim is extremely obese: she is five foot two and weighs over 350 pounds. Her diagnostic tests revealed hypothyroidism. Her cholesterol levels were normal, but her blood sugar was slightly elevated, as was her cortisol level.

We worked on all those health issues, and by her fifth visit, Kim felt her self-esteem was being restored. And now that she feels more confident she's not really sure she even wants to save her marriage. She wants to feel and look great for herself.

Recommended supplements: *EGCG*, to boost fat burning; *chromium*, for her slightly elevated blood sugar; *5-HTP*, to help with her mild depression and anxiety, and to help control appetite; *chitosan*, to reduce the absorption of fat, since Kim really likes fatty foods.

CLA (CONJUGATED LINOLEIC ACID)

"CLA is not only good for overweight, but may help reduce many risk factors for chronic disease, like high cholesterol, high triglycerides, glucose intolerance, and a family history of cancer," says Dr. Born. "I also recommend it for people who have a goal of losing *inches* as well as pounds, because CLA improves body composition, increasing muscle and decreasing fat."

Consider taking CLA if . . .

- You have difficulty with diet and exercise regimens, but still want to lose fat and gain muscle.

- You want to keep your weight stable.

- You want to prevent weight regain after a diet.

- You feel depressed when you diet.

- You want to lose fat after pregnancy.

- You are perimenopausal or menopausal and want to prevent fat gain or lose fat.

- You want to prevent osteoporosis.

- You have risk factors for heart disease or diabetes, or a family history of cancer.

BARBARA: Perimenopausal—and worried about weight gain
CLA, BCAA

Dr. Connealy: Barbara is a thirty-six-year-old, high-powered attorney from Japan. She's single, doesn't have any children, and has been focusing on her career since her boyfriend was killed in an auto accident five years ago. She's not depressed but admits to skipping meals. She enjoys running on the beach near her home every morning. She's five foot ten and weighs 128 pounds.

She's going to meet with our nutritionist, mainly for accountability (she occasionally indulges her sweet tooth) and to get advice and encouragement about eating a balanced diet.

Her Pap smear and physical are normal, and her blood pressure is good. Her lab work shows her to be perimenopausal (which means she is around the time of menopause). She is informed that due to the gradual decline of her hormones she will begin to lose muscle mass, and will need to add weight-bearing exercise.

For her general health, I started her on natural hormone replacement therapy, omega-3 fatty acids, a comprehensive multivitamin for women, and calcium.

Recommended supplements: CLA, to keep her weight stable; *BCAA (branched-chain amino acids)*, to maintain her muscle mass.

HCA (HYDROXYCITRIC ACID)

"I've found HCA is effective in people who have a hard time sticking to diets, because it helps reduce appetite," says Dr. Born. "It can also help reduce body fat in people who find themselves slowly gaining weight, at the rate of 5 or 10 pounds a year."

Consider taking HCA if . . .

- You want help controlling appetite.

- You need help sticking with a low-calorie diet.

- You find yourself on a weight-loss "plateau" and just can't lose the last 5 or 10 pounds.

- You want to lose belly fat.

MARIA: Liposuction, but no results

HCA, chromium, soluble fiber

Dr. Connealy: Maria had liposuction a year ago, but she's very disappointed that it didn't result in any weight loss. She has a fifteen-year-old son and has been divorced for several years. She feels older than her age of forty-two.

She says she's constantly on the latest diet, but her eating habits don't reflect self-control. She's never hungry in the morning, but about three to four times a week she stops at Starbucks and gets a coffee mocha with an extra shot of espresso. By lunchtime, she's famished, and she races out of the office to the local fast-food restaurant, where she has her favorite pizza or a chili cheeseburger and an extra-large Diet Coke. Every day she feels tired about 3 P.M. and later drags herself home, where she eats popcorn or a frozen dinner or grabs some chips. Her weight in high school was about 115 pounds, her pregnancy weight about 142, and her current weight is 150. She's only five foot one and obese. She wants to stop the yo-yo dieting and eat for her health, not just for looks.

Maria will need frequent office visits with myself or another doctor, with a nutritionist, and perhaps with a counselor to encourage her to address the root of her overeating disorder. I ask her to take a daily multivitamin and omega-3 fatty acids.

Recommended supplements: *HCA*, to help control appetite and reduce body fat; *chromium*, to help blood sugar disordered by mochas, cola, and fast food, and to create more fat burning; a *soluble fiber supplement*, to help Maria feel fuller at meals, so she doesn't overeat as readily.

MCT (MEDIUM-CHAIN TRIGLYCERIDES)

MCT is very helpful in burning fat, says Dr. Born. She finds it particularly helpful in people on low-fat diets. "On those types of diets, the body senses it's in 'starvation mode' and stops burning fat. A healthy fat like MCT can help prevent this."

Consider taking MCT if . . .

- You don't want to regain the weight you've lost.

ROBERT: Thinning hairline, expanding waistline
MCT, EGCG

Dr. Connealy: Robert was referred to us by his wife, Kathleen. They've been married for three years. He's forty-six, and she's a very active twenty-nine-year-old woman who teaches volleyball at a local high school.

Robert is six foot two and weighs 215 pounds. Two and a half years ago he was lean and solid at 205 pounds, and he's now still somewhat muscular. However, he started a new business six months ago. He used to go to the gym regularly, and at his previous job he had a salad and a fresh juice at a nearby juice bar. Now, he's not able to find time to exercise and he grabs fast food for lunch. He's beginning to feel flabby and sluggish—he gets home long after his wife does and goes straight to bed—and he really wants to avoid additional weight gain. Also, he's become very irritable lately.

He agreed to see us as a birthday gift to his wife, and she was also present at his appointment. His blood pressure was 160/100, which is high, and his lab work was unremarkable, except for low levels of hormones such as DHEA and testosterone.

For his general health, I recommended a multi-ingredient nutrient and herbal formula for the prostate, a multivitamin for men, and omega-3 essential fatty acids.

Recommended supplements: Because he's not exercising but he doesn't want to gain weight, *MCT (medium-chain triglycerides)*, to increase calorie burning; *EGCG*, for increasing metabolism.

CHROMIUM

"I put every patient on chromium," says Dr. Born. This trace mineral improves insulin resistance and is a must for blood sugar control, she explains. The average dose she prescribes is 600 micrograms (mcg). "Most multivitamin and mineral supplements contain anywhere from 50 to 200 mcg, and that is not adequate for blood sugar control, particularly in someone with metabolic syndrome or diabetes." (Metabolic syndrome is a condition consisting of blood sugar problems, high triglycerides, high blood pressure, low HDL—and overweight. Dr. Born says that 90 percent of her patients with metabolic syndrome are low in chromium.)

"Chromium improves glucose levels, insulin levels, and all the measures of blood sugar metabolism," she says. "I use it in everyone who wants to lose weight."

Consider taking chromium if . . .

- You want to lose fat and gain muscle during a diet.

- You have insulin resistance.

- You have metabolic syndrome.

- You have type 2 diabetes.

- You are at risk for gestational diabetes.

- You take a steroid medication, like cortisone.

- You have type 1 diabetes.

MARISSA: She doesn't want to be on insulin
Chromium, carb blockers, EGCG

Dr. Connealy: Marissa has type 2 diabetes. She's on the maximum amount of oral medication that can be taken—and her blood sugar is still not controlled. Her family is from Mississippi and she was raised on soul food, and she wants me to understand that her family gets offended if she turns down the food she is offered every Sunday after church. Both of her parents and siblings are diabetic. Her father has kidney failure and has been getting dialysis for the past three years. He has been rushed to the hospital two times because of low blood pressure and electrolyte imbalances. She does not want to be on insulin like her parents. She wants to know what else she can do.

After reviewing her fasting lab work, I agree that she's at a critical juncture. She can do every last thing I tell her, and do it well, or prepare to die. She chooses to live. She said a prayer over her last Sunday meal with her family, asking for help in accomplishing her goals for health.

The program I recommend is a weekly appointment in our clinic, alternating between myself and our nutritionist. She is to keep a food and exercise journal. She is to reward herself at each positive milestone with something she really wants, like a new dress.

Recommended supplements: Chromium, 1,000 mcg a day, to help with insulin resistance; *carb blockers* before each meal, to help control the rise of blood sugar; *EGCG* three times a day, for anti-aging and other medicinal benefits.

CARBOHYDRATE INHIBITORS
(STARCH BLOCKERS AND SUGAR BLOCKERS)

"Americans are addicted to sugar and carbohydrates," says Dr. Connealy. "These supplements help control the rise of blood sugar after meals rich in carbohydrates, and therefore help insulin levels become more stable."

"They can also be used temporarily," says Dr. Born, "like when a person goes on a vacation or cruise and knows they'll be eating a lot of sugar."

Consider taking a carb blocker if . . .

- You love carbohydrates and want to eat them without guilt.

- You want to be on a low-carb diet, but not a strict one.

- You want better blood sugar control.

- You're about to eat a high-carb meal.

GREG: An obese teenager
Carb blockers, soluble fiber

Dr. Connealy: Greg is an obese teenager. He was initially seen in my office with both of his parents. I reviewed his family history, which includes diabetes, coronary artery disease, stroke, and sleep apnea. His parents are slightly overweight but not obese. Based on his bone structure and his parents' physical structure, I determined that Greg is 40 pounds overweight.

Greg is a freshman in high school, plays junior football, is a B-average student, and has many friends. His teachers would describe him as a very likable student, if sometimes a little too talkative.

For breakfast, Greg eats Cocoa Puffs with regular milk, and a piece of white toast with butter and jam. At lunchtime, he eats in the cafeteria, because no one in high school brings lunch from home. He couldn't remember what he had for lunch the day before, but it's usually pizza, chicken strips, or a cheeseburger and a soda. He doesn't eat any fresh fruits or vegetables. I asked Greg's parents about dinner, and they assured me that he eats well—so I asked what he had last night. They looked at each other, and I knew what the answer would be: "Well, we usually don't eat pizza, but we had a football game last night." More than likely, Greg will continue to eat poorly until his parents realize that they are part of the problem.

Recommended supplements: *Carb blockers* and a *fiber supplement,* to help Greg eat less and to control his blood sugar.

CHITOSAN AND OTHER SOLUBLE FIBERS

"I often recommend soluble fibers," says Dr. Born. "Not only do they help you feel fuller sooner, there is ample evidence that they can help balance blood sugar during the day, regulating appetite. They can also decrease LDL cholesterol, providing a double benefit to someone who is overweight with high cholesterol."

Consider taking chitosan or a mixed-fiber supplement if . . .

- You don't get enough fiber in your diet.

- You eat too much fat.

- You want to feel less hungry between meals.

- You want an option other than Xenical or Alli, drugs that inhibit fat absorption.

- You want to lower blood lipids, like cholesterol and triglycerides.

GRETA: Loves French fries, bacon-mushroom burgers, and strawberry shakes
Chitosan, chromium, EGCG

Dr. Connealy: Greta is a twenty-two-year-old college student. Although her grades were high enough for her to attend a university, her parents could not afford to send her and she's attending a local junior college. She drives the old family car, lives with her parents, and shares her room with her ten-year-old sister, Rebecca. Greta is five foot five and weighs 150 pounds. Rebecca is five foot seven and weighs 108 pounds.

For breakfast, they both eat oatmeal or sugar-free cereal with 2 percent milk. Greta has a part-time job at a local restaurant, where she usually eats her lunch. She loves French fries and bacon-mushroom burgers with a strawberry shake—and besides, she feels she deserves it.

Her parents accompany her to her first appointment. Her blood tests reveal that she has prediabetes—and she is shocked. This condition can be controlled with healthy eating and exercise. Ideally, Greta would get adequate fiber and nutrients from a diet rich in fruits and vegetables. But, realistically that might not be possible for her right now, so we agree to compromise—she *will* use the supplement program I recommend.

Recommended supplements: *Chitosan*, for fat blocking and fiber; *chromium*, for prediabetes; *EGCG*, for general health.

5-HTP (5-HYDROXY-L-TRYPTOPHAN)

"In our clinics, we use serotonin-boosting 5-HTP for very obese patients who are 100 to 150 pounds overweight, people who typically have many of the problems that can accompany extreme obesity, like insomnia, chronic headaches, depression, and fibromyalgia," says Dr. Born. "And, in fact, when we check urine levels for serotonin, typically 95 percent of obese patients are low in this important neurotransmitter."

Consider taking 5-HTP if . . .

- You crave and overeat carbohydrates.

- You are overweight and have other health problems reflecting low levels of serotonin, such as depression and insomnia.

JANET: She's addicted to sugar and carbs—even after heart surgery
5-HTP, chromium, L-arabinose (sugar blocker)

Dr. Connealy: Janet is a fifty-seven-year-old single mother who came to our clinic seeking to lose weight. She is five foot four and currently weighs 189 pounds. She has an elevated BMI, high cholesterol, high blood pressure, and a history of diabetes during pregnancy. She lacks the motivation to exercise and appears to be clinically depressed, but she says she plans to begin exercising at Curves, which opened near her job about a year ago. She's tired of being tired, and is eager to hear my suggestions.

I drew her fasting blood panel and had her return two weeks later to discuss her results and a plan of action. Her total cholesterol is 254, her LDL is 173, and her triglycerides are 588—all very high. Her blood sugar and insulin levels are also elevated, and she has microscopic blood in her urine, an indication of compromised kidney function. Because she has multiple risk factors for heart disease, I schedule her for a coronary heart scan. She reluctantly agrees.

Soon, I receive a call from Janet's cardiologist: her right coronary artery is 50 percent blocked and her left coronary artery is 90 percent blocked. She is admitted to the cardiac intensive care unit for bypass surgery.

Janet comes to see me a few months after her surgery. She is on three different medications for her heart, one for her diabetes, and one for high cholesterol. She has lost 5 pounds, which she attributes to stress. She has been exercising as part of her cardiac rehabilitation, but she's still craving carbohydrates—she admits that she's addicted to sugar and carbs.

I recommend a number of supplements for her general health, including a multivitamin, a B-complex vitamin, and omega-3 fatty acids.

Recommended supplements: 5-HTP, for sugar cravings and anxiety; *chromium*, 1,000 mcg, 500 in the morning and 500 in the evening, for elevated blood sugar; the sugar blocker *L-arabinose*, because of elevated triglycerides. (When the system is overloaded with sugar, it is converted into triglycerides.)

HMB AND BCAA (HYDROXY METHYLBUTYRATE AND BRANCHED-CHAIN AMINO ACIDS)

"HMB helps increase strength during intense exercise, and BCAA helps preserve muscle mass," says Dr. Connealy.

FINDING A SUPPLEMENT-SAVVY DOCTOR

You go to your doctor to talk about weight-loss supplements, tell him you've decided to take chromium and would like his help monitoring your intake and your blood sugar levels, and he says, "I'm not going to treat you if you decide to take chromium."

Perhaps you should find another doctor.

"I recommend going to a doctor who balances conventional and integrative treatments," says Tammy L. Born, DO. "You don't want to see a doctor who says that he won't treat you because your preferences don't fit his paradigm. That's a doctor who cares more about his paradigm than his patients."

What type of doctor should a person interested in weight-loss supplements look for? "Find a doctor with whom you can communicate," says Dr. Born. "A person who can take into account *all* the factors of your life. Someone who is caring and looks at the whole person, not just you as a 'weight-loss patient'—but as someone who has many issues that need to be addressed."

PROFESSIONAL ASSOCIATIONS

The following professional associations are good places to start in a search for a doctor who would likely be knowledgeable about and supportive of the use of supplements for weight loss:

Consider taking HMB or BCAA if . . .

- You exercise intensively and want to avoid soreness and muscle loss.

- You're over thirty-five and want to avoid gradual, age-related muscle loss.

- You're over sixty-five and want to slow or even stop sarcopenia, the loss of muscle mass associated with old age.

American College for the Advancement of Medicine (ACAM). Founded in 1973, this 1,000-member organization is a not-for-profit medical society dedicated to educating physicians and other health care professionals on the latest findings and emerging procedures in preventive and nutritional medicine. Their Web site, at www.acam.org, includes a search function to find an ACAM member in your area, and is also searchable by specialties.

International College of Integrative Medicine. This is a group of 130 doctors dedicated to complementary medicine. Their site, at www.icimed.com, includes a search function for finding a member in your area.

American Holistic Medical Association. The mission of the AHMA is to support practitioners in their personal and professional development as healers and to educate physicians about holistic medicine. Their Web site, at www.holisticmedicine.org, allows you to search for a holistic practitioner in your area.

The American Association of Naturopathic Physicians. Naturopathic medicine combines safe and effective traditional therapies with the most current advances in modern medicine. In addition to the basic medical sciences and conventional diagnostics, naturopathic physicians (NDs) are trained in a broad range of naturopathic medical modalities, including therapeutic nutrition, herbal medicine, homeopathy, classical Chinese medicine, and hydrotherapy. This 1,800-member organization consists only of NDs who are licensed or eligible to be licensed as primary care providers. Their site, at www.naturopathic.org, includes a search function for finding a licensed naturopathic physician in your area.

STEVE: Help for twice-a-day training
HMB

Dr. Connealy: Steve is a tall, lean, good-looking redhead (who also happens to be proud he's Irish). He is a very successful architectural engineer with a lovely wife who home schools their two boys. He's been treated for Stage 1 melanoma with complete success.

He sets his alarm to reapply his sunblock with SPF 60 every three hours during the day; has a computer printout of his meals and their caloric, fiber, and sodium values; and he flosses his teeth after every meal. He goes to the gym twice a day—at 4:30 A.M. and 1 P.M.

He inherited high triglycerides from his mother's side of the family; otherwise, he assures me he is in perfect health. He would like to monitor his cholesterol and lipids, and his chemistry panels, for which he has kept detailed records for the past twenty years. And he will accept any recommendations I offer provided that I immediately send his results to him, instead of his having to see me for follow-up visits to discuss them.

I agree to send Steve's results to him, and I advise him to take a multivitamin, omega-3 essential fatty acids, extra vitamin C for his immune system, selenium, saw palmetto and lycopene for his prostate, and green tea because of his history of cancer and elevated triglycerides.

Recommended supplements: *HMB*, to increase his strength during his exhaustive, twice-a-day training session, and to increase his lean body mass.

PART IX

Natural Fat Loss Plus

Easy Calorie Control
Forget About Carbs, Fat, and Protein: The Secret to Weight Loss Is Calorie-Wise Satisfaction

If you've been on lots of diets, you might feel like you've been eating in the middle of a three-ring circus—with you as the frowning and frantic clown.

Ladies and gentlemen, in this ring we have the *low-fat* diet. Don't touch that butter! In this ring, the *low-carb* diet—pass the butter! And in this ring, the *high-protein diet*—let's all lose weight on filet mignon!

Maybe you've gone on a diet that promotes the importance of a particular *macronutrient*: carbohydrate, fat, or protein. Or a diet that tells you to *balance* all three. Or a diet that tells you to pay attention to "good" and "bad" carbs/fats/proteins, as if you had angel food cake whispering to you from one shoulder and deviled ham perched on the other. Maybe you felt as though you were trying to juggle three macronutrients. And maybe—like 95 percent of dieters—you dropped the ball.

Well, we talked to several top dieticians and nutritionists who have spent decades helping people lose weight. They've seen macronutrient-based diet fads come and go (and come again and go again). And here's what they're saying to their carb-confused, fat-flustered, and protein-puzzled clients:

It's time to take a vacation from the Macronutrient Circus. Because it's not just the carbs. It's not just the fat. It's not just the protein. It's mostly the *calories*.

SOLVING THE CALORIE EQUATION

There is no macronutrient "trick" to weight loss. For most people, gaining or losing weight is a matter of metabolic mathematics, a "calorie equation" as unvarying as $1+1 = 2$.

- If you eat more calories than you burn, you gain weight.

- If you burn more calories than you eat, you lose weight.

But counting those calories seems like such a . . . well, such a pain in the place where you wish fewer calories were camping out. We've got good nutritional news for you.

We already told you some of the good news: you don't have to worry a whole lot about keeping track of macronutrients. The better news: controlling calories is a simple, straightforward, and effective way to lose weight. The best news: you don't have to go on a diet to do it.

Yes, calorie control isn't about dieting. It's about learning a *lifestyle*—an easy and enjoyable way to eat that doesn't involve daily deprivation. In fact, calorie control can be as easy as brushing your teeth or taking a shower.

And because you're an individual—because no one lifestyle fits all lives—we're presenting you with a variety of approaches to easy calorie control. Like our advice about taking the weight-loss supplements in this book, we think the best approach to calorie control is *customized*: familiarize yourself with the possibilities, and then pick the approach that appeals to you.

To get you started, we teamed up with Tracy Gensler, a registered dietician from Washington, DC, and author of *The Anti-Aging Fitness Prescrip-*

tion, to create the Natural Fat-Loss Pharmacy Meal Plan—a month's worth of healthy breakfasts, lunches, dinners, and snacks that will help you lose weight. It's perfect for people who hate counting calories (who doesn't?)—but who know that calories count!

THE NATURAL FAT-LOSS PHARMACY MEAL PLAN

To lose weight, most women should eat between 1,200 and 1,500 calories per day and most men between 1,500 and 1,800 calories—that's why we've made 1,500 the total number of calories in the Natural Fat-Loss Pharmacy Meal Plan. This level of calories will help you feel full after you eat, have the energy to get through a demanding day's worth of work and play, and meet daily nutritional goals.

But as we said earlier, you don't have to *count* those calories. The meal plan provides 30 days of healthy breakfasts, lunches, dinners, and snacks tailored to the perfect calorie count. You can eat the meals according to "plan"—on the first day, enjoy the Day 1 breakfast, Day 1 lunch, Day 1 dinner, and Day 1 snack, and so on for 30 days. Or you can mix and match the recipes if you prefer. For example, you can select the Day 1 breakfast, Day 10 lunch, Day 20 dinner, and Day 30 snack, or any other combination, to automatically get a total of 1,500 calories every day. You'll also get a good sampling of healthy foods like fruits and vegetables, whole grains, lean protein, low-fat dairy products, and unsaturated fats (including heart-healthy omega-3 fats). And no matter how you combine the recipes, each day on the Natural Fat-Loss Pharmacy Meal Plan also supplies you with filling and healthy proportions of carbohydrates, protein, fat, and fiber.

Some folks may need slightly more calories, including avid exercisers (who need fuel for workouts) and larger men (who can eat more than 1,500 calories and still lose weight). If you're in one of these categories, you'll find suggestions for adding extra calories with one of our 300-Calorie Super Snacks (page 301).

What can you drink with your meals, other than water? Focus on low-cal liquids, like fat-free cow's milk, 1% cow's milk, light chocolate soy milk, light vanilla soy milk, or plain low-fat soy milk (amounts are provided with the recipes). And help yourself to unlimited refills of coffee, tea, and flavored seltzers. (For seltzers, make sure "natural flavoring" is the only added ingredient.) Try to stay away from calorie-dense drinks, like full-fat milk, soft drinks, and fruit juices. As for water itself: Plan on drinking at least six 8-ounce glasses of water every day. That will help you feel fuller during the day—and refreshed!

Better Breakfasts

If you're trying to lose weight, eating a healthy breakfast is a must. Studies show that breakfast-eaters consume fewer calories throughout the day and are less likely to succumb to late-day overeating. Each breakfast in the Natural Fat-Loss Pharmacy Meal Plan provides 350 calories. You'll find options for eating in, eating out, or taking your breakfast with you. If you prefer to repeat a few of your favorite breakfasts rather than sampling a new one every day, go right ahead!

Day 1 Breakfast. Crunchy Yogurt with Fruit and Nuts

In a serving bowl, top 6 ounces plain low-fat yogurt with ½ cup Kashi Good Friends cereal, ½ cup frozen seedless grapes (freeze the grapes for at least 1 hour), and 2 tablespoons chopped peanuts.

Day 2 Breakfast. Tomato and Mozzarella Wrap

Preheat the oven to 250°F. Place one (8") whole wheat soft tortilla (such as a Flatout brand Healthy Grains wrap or a soft tortilla with 140 calories and at least 4 grams fiber) in a baking dish and top it with 1 chopped tomato mixed with 1 teaspoon chopped fresh basil (or ½ teaspoon dried basil) and 1 teaspoon extra-virgin olive oil. Sprinkle that with 1 ounce reduced-fat shredded mozzarella cheese. Bake for 3 to 4 minutes, or until the cheese is melted. Serve with 1 cup fat-free milk for drinking.

Day 3 Breakfast. Whole Grain Waffles with Apple and Walnuts

In a small bowl, combine 1 finely chopped medium apple, 1 tablespoon chopped walnuts, and ⅛ teaspoon cinnamon. Toast 2 whole grain frozen waffles, such as Kashi GOLEAN Original, and top them evenly with the apple mixture. Serve with 1 cup light vanilla soy milk for drinking.

Day 4 Breakfast. Cranberry Pita

In a small bowl, combine 3 ounces plain low-fat yogurt, 1 ounce soft goat cheese, and 1 teaspoon dried cranberries. Spread one (6½") whole wheat pita with the yogurt mixture. Serve with ½ cup light chocolate soy milk for drinking.

Day 5 Breakfast. Bran Muffin with Café au Lait

Warm one (3" diameter, 2" high) bran muffin—check the label for about 160 calories, 3 grams fiber, and 0 grams trans fats. In a large cup, combine 1 cup brewed coffee, 1 cup fat-free milk, and 2 teaspoons vanilla-flavored (or your favorite flavor) coffee creamer. Heat in a microwave oven on high power for 30 seconds. Have the muffin and café au lait with 1 small pear.

Day 6 Breakfast. Almond Butter and Apricot Sandwich

Toast 1 slice of whole wheat bread, such as Healthy Choice Hearty 100% Whole Grain, and cut it in half. Spread one half with 1 tablespoon almond butter and top it with 4 dried apricot halves and the other half of the bread slice. Have the sandwich with 1 cup fat-free milk for drinking.

Day 7 Breakfast. Smoothie with an English Muffin

To make the smoothie, in a blender, combine 1 cup fresh or frozen unsweetened raspberries (if using frozen raspberries, don't thaw them for a really thick, frosty smoothie), 1 cup plain low-fat yogurt, and 6 tablespoons calcium-fortified orange juice and blend until smooth. Serve it with half a toasted whole grain English muffin (at least 3 grams fiber) spread with 2 teaspoons light, trans-fat-free margarine.

Day 8 Breakfast. Peanut Banana Wrap

Open one (8") whole wheat soft tortilla (such as a Flatout brand Healthy Grains wrap or a soft tortilla with 140 calories and at least 4 grams fiber). Lay 1 small peeled banana on the tortilla, sprinkle it with 1 tablespoon chopped peanuts, and roll it up to eat it. Serve with 1 cup fat-free milk for drinking.

Day 9 Breakfast. Peanut Butter Toast and Café au Lait

Toast 1 slice rye bread (at least 2 grams fiber) and spread with 1 tablespoon peanut butter. In a large cup, combine 1 cup light chocolate soy milk with 1 cup brewed coffee and heat in a microwave oven on high power for 30 seconds, if desired. Serve with 1 medium apple.

Day 10 Breakfast. Kiwifruit and Cottage Cheese Pita

Fill one (6½") whole wheat pita with ⅓ cup 1% or fat-free cottage cheese and 1 sliced kiwifruit. Serve with 1 cup fat-free milk.

Day 11 Breakfast. Honey Nut Ricotta Cereal Bowl

In a serving bowl, combine ½ cup low-fat ricotta cheese, 2 tablespoons chopped walnuts, 1 tablespoon maple syrup, 1 teaspoon honey, and ⅛ teaspoon ground cinnamon; mix well. Stir in ½ cup Kashi Good Friends cereal or ½ cup Cheerios (or 60 calories' worth of your favorite high-fiber cereal).

Day 12 Breakfast. Cherry-Almond Cream Cereal

Toast 1 tablespoon slivered almonds in a dry, heavy skillet over low heat, stirring constantly, for about 1 minute; do not let them burn. In a serving bowl, combine 1 cup plain low-fat yogurt and ¾ cup Kashi Heart to Heart cereal or 1 cup Barbara's Bakery GrainShop cereal. Stir in the toasted almonds and 1 tablespoon dried cherries.

Day 13 Breakfast. Easy Apple Pecan Cobbler

In a microwaveable bowl, combine ⅓ cup low-fat granola (choose granola without raisins), 1 chopped medium apple, 2 tablespoons calcium-fortified orange juice, 1 tablespoon chopped pecans, and ¼ teaspoon grated orange peel. Heat in a microwave oven on high power for 3 minutes, then let stand for 1 minute. Top with 1 tablespoon light sour cream. Serve with 1 cup light vanilla soy milk for drinking.

Day 14 Breakfast. Vanilla Bean Cereal Bowl

In a serving bowl, combine 1 cup plain low-fat yogurt with ¼ teaspoon pure vanilla extract. Add ½ cup Kashi Good Friends cereal or ½ cup Cheerios (or 60 calories' worth of your favorite high-fiber cereal), 1 sliced medium banana, and 1 tablespoon slivered almonds; stir well.

Day 15 Breakfast. Peanut Butter and Chocolate Crunch

In a microwaveable bowl, combine 1 tablespoon mini chocolate chips and 1 tablespoon peanut butter. Heat in a microwave oven on high power for 30 seconds. Add ½ cup Kashi Heart to Heart cereal or 1 cup Barbara's Bakery GrainShop cereal and stir well. Serve with 1 cup light chocolate soy milk for drinking.

Day 16 Breakfast. Tropical Mueslix

In a serving bowl, combine ¾ cup mueslix, such as Kellogg's Mueslix, with ½ cup fat-free milk and ½ cup cubed pineapple (canned in juice or water or fresh). Serve with 1 cup fat-free milk for drinking.

Day 17 Breakfast. Chunky Peanut Oatmeal

Make the oatmeal according to the package directions using ½ cup old-fashioned rolled oats and ½ cup light plain soy milk. Top with 1 tablespoon chopped peanuts. Serve with 1 cup light plain soy milk for drinking.

Day 18 Breakfast. Hearty Pecan and Raisin Grits

Prepare 1 instant packet (½ cup dry) grits following the package directions, using ½ cup fat-free milk. Stir in 1 tablespoon wheat germ, 1 tablespoon chopped pecans, and 1 tablespoon raisins. Serve with 1 cup fat-free milk for drinking.

Day 19 Breakfast. Cinnamon Almond Granola

In a microwaveable bowl, combine ⅓ cup low-fat granola cereal, such as Kellogg's, with 1 chopped medium apple and 2 tablespoons slivered almonds. Sprinkle with ⅛ teaspoon ground cinnamon, then add 1 cup fat-free milk. (For a thicker consistency, use ½ cup fat-free milk and drink the remaining ½ cup milk.) Heat the granola mixture in a microwave oven on high power for 60 to 90 seconds.

Day 20 Breakfast. Cherry Spoon Smoothie

In a blender, combine 1 cup fresh or frozen unsweetened pitted cherries (if using frozen cherries, don't thaw them for a really thick, frosty smoothie) and 1 cup plain low-fat yogurt; blend until smooth. Transfer to a serving bowl and top with ½ cup Kashi GOLEAN cereal (or 70 calories' worth of your favorite high-fiber cereal) and 1 tablespoon chopped pecans. Eat it with a spoon.

Day 21 Breakfast. Diner Swiss-Veggie Omelet (*Dine-Out Option*)

At your favorite family restaurant, order an egg-white veggie omelet (ask the server to use 4 egg whites or ½ cup egg substitute, and request that no oil be used in cooking) with 1 ounce Swiss cheese and any vegetables you'd like, such as bell peppers, onions, tomatoes, or mushrooms. Eat with 1 slice of whole wheat toast spread with 2 teaspoons jam and topped with ½ cup mixed fruits.

Day 22 Breakfast. Creamy Strawberry Smoothie

In a blender, combine 1½ cups fresh or frozen unsweetened strawberries (if using frozen berries, don't thaw for a really thick, frosty smoothie), 1 cup fat-free milk, 4 ounces firm tofu made with calcium sulfate, ⅓ cup calcium-fortified orange juice, and ¼ teaspoon vanilla extract and blend until smooth. Transfer it to a serving bowl and top with 2 tablespoons low-fat granola cereal, such as Kellogg's (without raisins). Eat it with a spoon.

Day 23 Breakfast. Veggie Sausage Scramble

In a microwave oven, heat 1 veggie sausage patty (80 calories maximum) according to the package directions; crumble the patty and set it aside. In a medium skillet, heat ½ teaspoon canola oil over medium heat. Add ¼ cup chopped onion and cook for 2 to 3 minutes, or until the onion just begins to soften. Add 2 lightly beaten egg whites and the crumbled veggie patty and cook for 1 to 2 minutes, or until the eggs are set. Serve with 1 cup fresh or frozen unsweetened raspberries mixed with 6 ounces plain low-fat yogurt.

Day 24 Breakfast. Cheesy Vegetable Toast

In a medium skillet, heat ½ teaspoon extra-virgin olive oil over medium heat. Add ¼ cup chopped green bell pepper, ¼ cup sliced white mushrooms, and ⅛ teaspoon onion powder and cook, stirring, for 3 to 4 minutes, or until the vegetables are just softened. Stir in ⅓ cup shredded reduced-fat mozzarella cheese and heat just until melted. Spoon the mixture over 1 slice rye toast and serve with 1 sliced orange and 1 cup fat-free milk for drinking.

Day 25 Breakfast. Blueberry French Toast

In a medium bowl, whisk together 1 egg white and 2 tablespoons fat-free milk. In a medium skillet, melt 1 tablespoon light, trans-fat-free margarine over medium heat. Dip 1 slice whole wheat bread into the egg mixture and add it to the pan. Sprinkle the bread with ⅛ teaspoon ground cinnamon and cook until the egg is set on the bottom. Turn the bread over and cook until the egg is set on the other side. Top with 1 cup fresh or frozen unsweetened blueberries and 1 tablespoon chopped walnuts. Serve with 1 cup fat-free milk for drinking.

Day 26 Breakfast. Greek-Style Egg White Scramble

Pierce one 3-ounce potato a few times with a fork. Cook the potato in a microwave oven on high power for 3 to 4 minutes, or until tender. Allow the potato to cool briefly, then cut it into ¼" chunks. In a small bowl, whisk to-gether 2 egg whites and ¼ cup fat-free milk. In a medium skillet, heat ½ tea-spoon extra-virgin olive oil over medium heat. Add the egg-white mixture and potato and stir. Immediately add 1 cup fresh stemmed spinach leaves and ½ ounce feta cheese and cook, stirring, until the eggs are set. Serve with 1 cup fresh or frozen unsweetened blackberries and 1 cup fat-free milk for drinking.

Day 27 Breakfast. Waffles with Strawberries

Toast 2 whole grain waffles, such as Kashi GOLEAN Original. Top with 6 ounces plain low-fat yogurt mixed with 1½ cups fresh or frozen unsweet-ened strawberries.

Day 28 Breakfast. Bagel Shop (*Dine-Out Option*)

At your bagel shop, order half of a whole wheat, granola, or cinnamon raisin bagel. Have it topped with a 1-ounce slice of American, Muenster, or Swiss cheese, and lettuce, tomato, and onion, if you'd like. Cut it in half to make a bagel sandwich. Serve with one (12-ounce) fat-free latte. (Take the other half of the bagel home.)

Day 29 Breakfast. Maple Almond Blackberry Bowl

In a serving bowl, combine 1 cup fresh or frozen unsweetened blackberries with 1 cup plain low-fat yogurt, ½ cup Kashi Heart to Heart cereal or 1 cup Barbara's Bakery GrainShop cereal, and 2 teaspoons maple syrup. Top with 1 tablespoon slivered almonds.

Day 30 Breakfast. Pecan-Topped Waffle

Toast 1 whole grain waffle, such as Kashi GOLEAN Original. Spread with 2 teaspoons light, trans-fat-free margarine and sprinkle with 1 tablespoon chopped pecans. Serve with ½ cup fresh or frozen unsweetened raspberries and 2 cups fat-free milk for drinking.

Luscious Lunches

When it comes to losing weight, lunchtime is often crunch time—unless you plan ahead, you're likely to opt for fast food or something out of the vending machine. Instead, rely on the 30 days of lower-calorie lunches from the Natural Fat-Loss Pharmacy Meal Plan. These delicious meals will help you feel full (but not stuffed). And because they emphasize slowly digested, healthy foods, you'll avoid a late-afternoon drop in blood sugar—the main cause of midafternoon fatigue and the sugary snacking that often goes with it. Each lunch delivers 450 calories. As with breakfast, eat according to the plan, or pick any day's lunch that looks tasty. And don't worry about repeating favorites. Your choices include meals you can prepare in advance and take along with you and options for eating out.

Day 1 Lunch. Ginger Chicken with Whole Wheat Couscous
In a large zipper-lock bag, combine 4 tablespoons calcium-fortified orange juice, 2 teaspoons reduced-sodium soy sauce, and ½ teaspoon each minced garlic and ground ginger. Add 3 ounces boneless, skinless chicken breast, turn it to coat it well, and marinate it in the refrigerator for at least 30 minutes or overnight. In a medium skillet, heat 1 teaspoon extra-virgin olive oil over medium heat. Add the chicken and marinade and cook for 3 to 4 minutes per side, or until cooked through. Serve with ½ cup cooked whole wheat couscous mixed with 1 chopped tomato and 1 teaspoon extra-virgin olive oil.

Day 2 Lunch. Chinese Chicken and Vegetable Stir-Fry
In a microwave oven, heat 3 Boca meatless Chik'n Nuggets or 1 Tyson low-fat Chicken Patty according to the package directions; cut into ¼" pieces and set aside. In a large skillet, heat 1 teaspoon sesame oil over medium heat. Add 2 cups Chinese-style frozen vegetables (such as bok choy, broccoli, carrots, water chestnuts) or any mixed vegetables and cook, stirring frequently,

for 4 to 5 minutes. Add ¾ cup cooked brown rice, 1 tablespoon rice vinegar, 1 tablespoon sesame seeds, 1 teaspoon reduced-sodium soy sauce, and the reserved chicken. Continue to cook, stirring frequently, for another 2 minutes, or until heated through.

Day 3 Lunch. Beans and Onion Spread on Whole Wheat Crackers

In a medium bowl, combine 1¼ cups rinsed and drained canned pinto beans, ¼ cup chopped onion, 1 tablespoon balsamic vinegar, 2 teaspoons extra-virgin olive oil, 1 teaspoon lemon juice, and ½ teaspoon minced garlic; toss well. Serve with 10 whole wheat trans-fat-free crackers (120 calories).

Day 4 Lunch. Chicken Caesar

In a large zipper-lock bag, combine 2 tablespoons lemon juice and ½ teaspoon dried dill. Add 4 ounces boneless, skinless chicken breast to the bag, turn it to coat it, and marinate it in the refrigerator for at least 30 minutes or overnight. While the chicken is marinating, make the croutons: Toast 2 slices pumpernickel bread and spread each slice with 2 teaspoons light, trans-fat-free margarine. Sprinkle each with ⅛ teaspoon dried basil. Cut the bread into ¼" cubes; set them aside. Coat a medium skillet with cooking spray and heat over medium heat. Add the chicken and marinade and cook for 3 to 4 minutes per side, or until the chicken is cooked through; let it cool briefly, then cut it into bite-size pieces. Place 3 cups romaine lettuce in a serving bowl. Add the chicken, 2 tablespoons light Caesar dressing (or 80 calories' worth of your favorite dressing), and 1 tablespoon Parmesan cheese; toss well. Top with the croutons.

Day 5 Lunch. Spicy Bean Dip with Pita Triangles

In a serving bowl, combine 1¼ cups fat-free refried beans, ¼ cup low-fat sour cream, 2 teaspoons extra-virgin olive oil, ¼ teaspoon chili powder, and ⅛ teaspoon dried cumin. Toast one (6") whole wheat pita and cut it into triangles to use for dipping.

Day 6 Lunch. Quick Mexican Tortilla

Fill one (8") whole wheat soft tortilla (such as a Flatout brand Healthy Grains wrap or a soft tortilla with 140 calories and at least 4 grams fiber) with ½ chopped avocado, ¼ cup shredded Cheddar cheese, ¾ cup sliced cucumber, and 2 tablespoons salsa. Serve with ½ cup blueberries.

Day 7 Lunch. Chickpea Dip with Tortilla Chips

In a serving bowl, combine ½ cup rinsed and drained canned chickpeas, ½ cup hummus, and 1 chopped tomato. Serve with 9 baked tortilla chips (about 0.5 ounce) for dipping.

Day 8 Lunch. Waldorf Salad

For the dressing, in a cup, combine ¼ cup plain low-fat yogurt, 1 tablespoon lemon juice, and ¼ teaspoon grated lemon peel. In a serving bowl, combine 3 cups spring mix greens, 1 cup seedless grapes, 1 chopped small apple, 2 chopped celery stalks, 2 tablespoons chopped walnuts, and 2 tablespoons golden raisins. Add the dressing and toss.

Day 9 Lunch. Grilled Vegetable Sandwich

In a medium skillet, heat 2 teaspoons extra-virgin olive oil over medium heat. Add ⅓ cup sliced green bell pepper, 1 chopped tomato, ¼ cup sliced white mushrooms, and ⅛ teaspoon each dried basil and dried oregano. Cook, stirring occasionally, until the vegetables are just softened, about 5 minutes. Meanwhile, toast 2 slices whole wheat bread, such as Healthy Choice Hearty 100% Whole Grain. Top 1 piece of toast with the vegetables and 1 slice light Swiss cheese; cover it with the remaining piece of toast. Serve with 1 sliced orange.

Day 10 Lunch. Honey Chicken with Brown Rice and Pine Nuts

In a large zipper-lock bag, combine 1 tablespoon lemon juice, 2 teaspoons honey, and 1 teaspoon reduced-sodium soy sauce. Add 3 ounces boneless, skinless chicken breast to the bag, turn it to coat it, and marinate it in the refrigerator for at least 30 minutes or overnight. Meanwhile, toast 1 teaspoon pine nuts in a heavy, dry skillet over medium heat for 1 minute, stirring constantly; do not let them burn. In a medium skillet, heat 1 teaspoon extra-virgin olive oil over medium heat. Add the chicken and marinade and cook for 3 to 4 minutes per side, or until the chicken is cooked through. Serve with ½ cup cooked brown rice topped with the toasted pine nuts. Follow with ½ cup plain low-fat yogurt topped with 1 cup fresh or frozen unsweetened raspberries.

Day 11 Lunch. Coleslaw with Apple and Walnuts
For the dressing, in a cup, combine ½ cup plain low-fat yogurt, 1 tablespoon light canola oil mayonnaise, 2 teaspoons white wine vinegar, 1 teaspoon honey, and ½ teaspoon poppy seeds; stir well. In a medium bowl, combine 2 cups prepared coleslaw (or 1 cup each shredded green and red cabbage and 2 tablespoons grated carrots) with 1 chopped medium apple and ¼ cup chopped walnuts. Add the dressing and toss.

Day 12 Lunch. Chef Salad with Whole Wheat Croutons
To make the croutons, toast 1 slice whole wheat bread and spread it with 2 teaspoons light, trans-fat-free margarine. Sprinkle it with ⅛ teaspoon dried basil. Cut the toast into ¼" cubes. In a serving bowl, combine 2 cups baby spinach leaves, 1 cup torn romaine lettuce, ¼ cup shredded reduced-fat mozzarella cheese, and 3 ounces deli ham sliced into strips. Toss with 2 tablespoons ranch dressing (or 85 calories' worth of your favorite dressing) and top with the croutons.

Day 13 Lunch. Black Bean Roll-Up
Top one (8") whole wheat soft tortilla (such as a Flatout brand Healthy Grains wrap or a soft tortilla with 140 calories and at least 4 grams fiber) with ½ cup cooked corn, ¼ cup rinsed and drained canned black beans, 3 tablespoons shredded Cheddar cheese, and 2 tablespoons salsa; roll it up. Serve with 1 cup fat-free milk for drinking.

Day 14 Lunch. Philly Beef on a Roll with a Berry Bowl

Open and toast (if desired) 1 whole wheat roll (about 150 calories and at least 2 grams fiber). Spread it with 1 tablespoon light canola oil mayonnaise. Top it with 3 ounces lean deli roast beef, such as Healthy Choice brand, 1 slice soy cheese, ¼ cup sliced onion, and ¼ cup sliced white mushrooms (if desired, cook the onion and mushrooms in a skillet lightly coated with cooking spray over low heat for 3 to 4 minutes, stirring frequently). Serve with 1 cup strawberries mixed with ½ cup blueberries.

Day 15 Lunch. Taco Salad

In a medium skillet, heat 2 teaspoons canola oil over medium heat. Add 3 ounces ground turkey breast and ⅛ teaspoon each dried cumin and chili powder. Cook, stirring, until turkey is cooked through, about 5 minutes. In a serving bowl, combine 2 cups torn romaine lettuce, ½ cup chopped red bell pepper, 2 tablespoons salsa, and the cooked turkey breast. Add 3 table-spoons feta cheese and 2 tablespoons regular salad dressing of your choice (about 85 calories' worth); toss well. Top with about 10 crumbled baked tortilla chips (0.5 ounce).

Day 16 Lunch. Mexican Wrap

In a medium skillet, heat 2 teaspoons canola oil over medium heat. Add 3 ounces 90% lean ground beef and sprinkle with a pinch of cayenne pepper. Cook, stirring, until the meat is cooked through, about 5 to 7 minutes. Fill one (8") whole wheat soft tortilla (such as a Flatout brand Healthy Grains wrap or a soft tortilla with 140 calories and at least 4 grams fiber) with the ground beef, ½ cup shredded romaine lettuce, 3 tablespoons light sour cream, and 2 tablespoons shredded Cheddar cheese. Serve with 1 sliced kiwifruit.

Day 17 Lunch. Tahini-Chickpea Pocket

Toast one (6½") whole wheat pita. Spread the inside with 2 tablespoons tahini or sesame butter. Fill the pita with ¼ cup sliced red bell pepper and ¼ cup rinsed and drained canned chickpeas.

Day 18 Lunch. Mediterranean Pasta

In a microwaveable dish, combine 1 cup cooked whole wheat pasta or Barilla Plus pasta (any shape), ½ cup spaghetti sauce, ½ cup cooked chopped leaf spinach, ¼ cup chopped red bell pepper, 3 tablespoons rinsed and drained canned white beans, and 2 tablespoons sliced black olives. Sprinkle with 1 tablespoon Parmesan cheese. Heat in a microwave oven on high power for 1 to 2 minutes. Follow with 1 cup grapes.

Day 19 Lunch. BBQ Chicken Salad

In a serving bowl, combine 3 cups shredded romaine lettuce, 4 ounces sliced deli chicken breast cut into small pieces, and ½ cup cooked corn. In a small bowl, combine ½ cup plain low-fat yogurt, 1 tablespoon barbeque sauce, 1 teaspoon white vinegar, and ½ teaspoon dried dill seed; stir well. Pour over salad and toss. Follow with 1 sliced mango.

Day 20 Lunch. Artichoke Pizza

Preheat the oven to 400°F. Place one (8") whole wheat thin pizza crust, such as a Boboli 100% Whole Wheat Thin Crust, on a baking sheet. Drizzle the crust with 1 teaspoon extra-virgin olive oil, then layer it with ½ cup fresh spinach leaves, 8 marinated artichoke hearts, and ⅓ cup chopped red onion. Sprinkle it with 1½ ounces goat cheese. Bake for 12 minutes, or until the crust starts to brown. Serve half of the pizza immediately and save the other half for the Day 23 lunch. The remaining pizza will keep in the refrigerator for up to 3 days, or it can be frozen for up to 1 month.

Day 21 Lunch. Pasta with Corn, Beans, and Tomato

In a medium bowl, combine 1½ cups cooked whole wheat pasta or Barilla Plus pasta (any shape) with ½ cup cooked corn, ½ cup rinsed and drained canned kidney beans, 1 chopped small tomato, 2 teaspoons extra-virgin olive oil, 2 teaspoons red wine vinegar, and 1 thinly sliced scallion; toss well.

Day 22 Lunch. Dijon Chicken Pita

Spread the inside of one (6½") whole wheat pita with 1 teaspoon Dijon mustard. Fill the pita with 3 ounces sliced chicken breast, 4 tablespoons shredded Cheddar cheese, and 2 tablespoons salsa. Sprinkle with black pepper.

Day 23 Lunch. Artichoke Pizza "Again"
Have the leftover half of the Artichoke Pizza from the Day 20 lunch. If you froze it, thaw it in the refrigerator overnight, then heat it in a 250°F oven for 10 to 12 minutes before serving.

Day 24 Lunch. Spinach Tuna Melt
Heat one (9-ounce) bag of frozen baby spinach in a microwave oven on high power for 2 minutes. Carefully transfer the hot spinach from the bag to a microwaveable bowl. Stir in 3 ounces rinsed and drained canned chunk light water-packed tuna and sprinkle with 1½ tablespoons Parmesan cheese. Place the bowl in the microwave oven and cook on high power for 30 to 45 seconds, or until the cheese begins to melt. Top with 15 halved grape tomatoes and ¼ cup dried sweetened cranberries.

Day 25 Lunch. Shrimp Cocktail with Broccoli and Cauliflower
In a large skillet, heat 2 teaspoons extra-virgin olive oil over medium heat. Add 4 ounces shelled and deveined uncooked medium shrimp. Cook, stirring, until the shrimp just turn pink, 2 to 3 minutes. Transfer the shrimp to a plate. In the same pan, heat another 2 teaspoons extra-virgin olive oil over medium heat. Add 1 cup each fresh or frozen broccoli and cauliflower florets and cook, stirring, just until softened, about 8 minutes. Sprinkle the cooked vegetables with ½ teaspoon crab-boil seasoning, if desired. Serve the vegetables with the shrimp and ¼ cup cocktail sauce for dipping. Follow with 1 sliced small apple and 1 sliced small pear.

Day 26 Lunch. Creamy Spinach and Bell Pepper Pasta
In a microwaveable bowl, combine 2 cups cooked whole wheat pasta or Barilla Plus pasta (any shape) with 2 cups fresh spinach leaves; ½ cup chopped red, orange, or yellow bell pepper; ½ cup fat-free ricotta cheese; and ¼ teaspoon minced garlic; stir well. Heat it in a microwave oven on high power

for 1½ to 2 minutes to warm it through, stirring once. Serve with 1 sliced mango (or 125 calories' worth of your favorite fruit).

Day 27 Lunch. Beef Vegetable Soup

Heat 2 cups canned vegetable beef soup, such as Campbell's Healthy Request Condensed Vegetable Beef, according to the package directions. Transfer the soup to a large serving bowl and top it with ¼ cup shredded reduced-fat mozzarella cheese. Toast 1 slice whole wheat bread and spread it with 2 teaspoons light, trans-fat-free margarine and serve it with the soup.

Day 28 Lunch. Grilled Cheese and Tomato Sandwich

Spread the outside of each of 2 slices whole wheat bread with 2 teaspoons light, trans-fat-free margarine. Fill the sandwich with 1 slice Swiss or American cheese and 1 thinly sliced small tomato. Coat a small skillet with cooking spray and heat it over medium heat. Grill the sandwich, turning once, until both sides are browned and the cheese is melted. Follow with 1½ cups grapes.

Day 29 Lunch. Salmon Caesar Salad (*Dine-Out Option*)

Order a salmon Caesar salad with light dressing on the side (eat about a palm-size amount of salmon and skip the croutons). With each forkful of salad, dip your fork into the dressing to keep your portion of salad dressing under 2 tablespoons. As a side dish, have a 3"-diameter crusty whole wheat or French roll. Follow with 1 small apple.

Day 30 Lunch. Pesto Chicken with Brown Rice

Toast ¼ cup slivered almonds in a dry, heavy skillet, stirring constantly, for about 2 minutes; do not let them burn. In a large zipper-lock bag, combine 1 tablespoon each lemon juice, red cooking wine, and Worcestershire sauce. Add 3 ounces boneless, skinless chicken breast, turn it to coat it, and marinate it in the refrigerator for at least 30 minutes or overnight. Meanwhile, make the pesto: In a food processor, combine the almonds, 1 tablespoon fresh basil leaves, 2 teaspoons extra-virgin olive oil, 1 clove garlic, and a pinch each of black pepper and nutmeg. Process until a coarse paste forms; set it aside. In a medium skillet, heat 2 teaspoons extra-virgin olive oil over medium heat. Add the chicken and cook for 4 to 5 minutes per side, or until cooked through. Top the chicken with the pesto sauce and serve it over ½ cup cooked brown rice.

Quick and Easy Dinners

The problem with dinnertime: It rolls around just when you've run out of energy for the day! You want to make something fast—and quick-to-prepare foods are often high in calories. Well, the dinners on the Natural Fat-Loss Pharmacy Meal Plan are all quick and easy to prepare *and* low in calories *and* delicious. With this plan, we think you'll look forward to making dinner every night. (And don't forget dessert! It's part of every dinner.) As with lunch, each meal is 450 calories. Feel free to mix and match meals, or repeat your favorites. Your choices for dinner include meals you can prepare in advance; frozen and ready-to-eat meals; and options for dining out.

Day 1 Dinner. Filet Mignon with Balsamic Spinach
Preheat the oven to 350°F. Coat a baking dish with cooking spray. Trim all visible fat from a 4-ounce filet mignon steak and make 6 to 8 tiny slices in the top. Place the beef in the baking dish, cut side up, and sprinkle the top with 1 tablespoon balsamic vinegar and ½ teaspoon each dried oregano and black pepper. Bake for 25 minutes. Meanwhile, in a medium skillet, heat 1 teaspoon extra-virgin olive oil over medium heat. Add ¼ cup chopped onion and cook, stirring, for 1 to 2 minutes. Add 2 cups baby spinach leaves, 1 tablespoon balsamic vinegar, and 1 minced clove garlic; continue to cook, stirring, for 2 minutes more, or until the spinach begins to wilt. Remove the pan from the heat and top the spinach mixture with 2 tablespoons feta cheese. Serve the vegetables with the beef. For dessert, have ¾ cup frozen grapes and 2 meringue cookies.

Day 2 Dinner. Quick Crispy Salmon Cakes with Corn
Preheat the oven to 350°F. Coat a baking dish with cooking spray. In a medium bowl, combine 3 ounces canned salmon with 3 tablespoons

seasoned bread crumbs, 1 tablespoon lemon juice, 1 tablespoon light canola oil mayonnaise, 1 egg white, 1 thinly sliced scallion, and ¼ teaspoon Dijon mustard. Form the mixture into 2 small patties, place them in the baking dish, and bake for 20 minutes, or until cooked through. Serve with 1 cooked ear sweet corn or ¾ cup cooked corn. Have 3 Hershey's Kisses for dessert.

Day 3 Dinner. Sweet Pork and Broccoli

Preheat the oven to 350°F. Coat a baking dish with cooking spray. Place one (3-ounce) pork tenderloin chop in the dish and top it with 2 teaspoons honey and ½ teaspoon brown sugar. Arrange 2 cups fresh or frozen broccoli florets around the pork, then add 2 tablespoons balsamic vinegar, 2 tablespoons calcium-fortified orange juice, 2 teaspoons extra-virgin olive oil, and 1 minced clove garlic. Top the broccoli with 1 thinly sliced small apple and bake for 35 minutes, or until the pork is cooked through. For dessert, have 1 fat-free Fudgsicle.

Day 4 Dinner. Weight Watchers Smart Ones Bistro Selections Stuffed Turkey Breast

Heat 1 serving of Weight Watchers Smart Ones Bistro Selections Stuffed Turkey Breast entrée according to the package directions (or choose any frozen entrée with 290 calories and less than 6 grams saturated fat). For dessert, have 1 small banana spread with 2 teaspoons peanut butter.

Day 5 Dinner. Baked Trout with Arugula Salad

Preheat the oven to 400°F. Coat a baking sheet with cooking spray. For the salad, in a serving bowl, combine 2 cups arugula, 2 tablespoons fresh or frozen unsweetened blueberries, and 2 tablespoons light salad dressing of your choice (about 80 calories). In a large zipper-lock bag, combine 1 ounce dry cornbread mix and 1 or 2 pinches each of cayenne pepper and black pepper. Add one (4-ounce) trout fillet and coat it well; transfer the trout to the baking sheet. Bake for 18 to 20 minutes, or until the trout is opaque and flakes easily with a fork. Serve the trout with the arugula salad. For dessert, have 1 frozen fruit juice bar (about 80 calories).

Day 6 Dinner. Two-Mustard Chicken with Bulgur

Preheat the oven to 350°F. Coat a baking dish with cooking spray. Place 3 ounces boneless, skinless chicken breast in the middle of the dish. In a cup, combine ½ teaspoon spicy brown mustard and ½ teaspoon Dijon mustard; brush the chicken with the mustard mixture. Arrange 10 medium asparagus spears around the chicken, drizzle them with 2 teaspoons extra-virgin olive oil, and sprinkle them with ¼ teaspoon each black pepper and dried thyme. Sprinkle the chicken and asparagus with 2 tablespoons Parmesan cheese. Bake for 20 to 22 minutes, or until the chicken is cooked through. Serve the chicken and asparagus over 1 cup cooked bulgur mixed with 1 chopped small tomato and a pinch of black pepper. For dessert, have 3 meringue cookies.

Day 7 Dinner. Mixed Vegetable Stir-Fry

In a medium skillet, heat 2 teaspoons sesame oil over medium heat. Add 1 cup frozen shelled edamame, ½ cup each broccoli and cauliflower florets, and ⅓ cup each sliced green and red bell peppers. Sprinkle the mixture with 1 tablespoon reduced-sodium soy sauce. Cook, stirring, until the vegetables are the desired crispness. Have 1 fat-free Fudgsicle for dessert.

Day 8 Dinner. Salmon and Zucchini

Preheat the oven to 350°F. Coat a baking dish with cooking spray. Place one (3-ounce) fillet of salmon in the middle of the dish. Surround the salmon with 1 sliced small zucchini. Sprinkle the zucchini with ⅛ teaspoon black pepper and bake for 15 minutes. Remove the dish from the oven and drizzle the zucchini and salmon with 2 tablespoons light ranch dressing. Return the dish to the oven and cook for 3 to 4 minutes more, or until the salmon is opaque and flakes easily with a fork. Serve with two (1-ounce) whole wheat dinner rolls, each spread with 1 teaspoon light, trans-fat-free margarine. For dessert, have 3 Hershey's Kisses.

Day 9 Dinner. Sesame Baked Chicken with Mango Brown Rice

Preheat the oven to 400°F. Coat a small baking dish with cooking spray. In a large zipper-lock bag, combine 1 tablespoon sesame seeds, 1 tablespoon whole wheat flour, and ⅛ teaspoon black pepper. Add 3 ounces boneless, skinless chicken breast and shake to coat it. Transfer the chicken to the baking dish and bake for 18 to 20 minutes, or until cooked through. Serve with ½ cup cooked brown rice mixed with 1 chopped small mango. For dessert, have a frozen fruit juice bar (about 80 calories).

Day 10 Dinner. Pork Barbeque with Corn
Coat a medium saucepan with cooking spray and heat it over medium heat. Add 2 tablespoons chopped white onion and cook, stirring, for 2 minutes. Add 2 teaspoons Worcestershire sauce, cover, and cook for 1 minute. Add 3 ounces ground pork tenderloin and 2 tablespoons low-sodium chicken broth; cook, uncovered, for 2 minutes, stirring frequently. Add 1 chopped tomato and 1 tablespoon barbeque sauce, cover, and continue to cook until the pork is cooked through, about 2 minutes more. Serve with ½ cup cooked corn. For dessert, have 2 meringue cookies.

Day 11 Dinner. Rosemary Chicken with Spicy Beans
Preheat the oven to 350°F. Sprinkle one (3-ounce) boneless, skinless chicken thigh with ¼ teaspoon rosemary and bake for 20 minutes, or until it is cooked through. In a microwaveable bowl, combine 1 cup rinsed and drained canned vegetarian beans with 1 tablespoon barbeque sauce and 1 teaspoon Dijon mustard. Heat the beans in a microwave oven on high power for 45 seconds, or until they are heated through. Serve with ½ cup cooked carrots topped with 1 teaspoon light, trans-fat-free margarine. For dessert, have 1 fat-free Fudgsicle.

Day 12 Dinner. Shrimp Salad with Whole Wheat Croutons
In a large zipper-lock bag, combine 3 ounces shelled and deveined medium shrimp with 3 tablespoons fat-free creamy Italian salad dressing; turn the shrimp to coat them and marinate them in the refrigerator for 10 minutes. Meanwhile, make the croutons: Toast 2 slices whole wheat bread, such as Healthy Choice Hearty 100% Whole Grain. Spread them with 2 teaspoons light, trans-fat-free margarine and sprinkle with ⅛ teaspoon dried basil. Cut

the toast into ¼" cubes. Coat a medium skillet with cooking spray and heat over medium heat. Add the shrimp and cook, stirring, for 2 to 3 minutes, or until the shrimp turn pink. In a serving bowl, toss the shrimp with 2 cups torn romaine lettuce, 1 tablespoon red wine vinegar, and 2 teaspoons extra-virgin olive oil. Top the salad with the croutons. For dessert, have 2 Hershey's Kisses.

Day 13 Dinner. Tomato Soup and Hearty Antipasto Salad

Heat 1 cup canned tomato soup, such as Campbell's Low Sodium Tomato Soup with Tomato Pieces (160 calories), according to the package directions. For the salad, combine 2 cups torn romaine lettuce, 5 chopped black olives, 1 ounce lean ham cut into strips, 2 tablespoons shredded mozzarella cheese, and 2 tablespoons light Italian dressing. Serve the soup with or followed by the salad. For dessert, have 1 Skinny Cow Ice Cream Sandwich (about 140 calories).

Day 14 Dinner. Honeydew Chicken Salad

In a serving bowl, combine 1 cup cubed honeydew, 3 ounces chopped roasted chicken breast, ½ cup plain low-fat yogurt, 2 chopped celery stalks, 1 thinly sliced scallion, and 2 teaspoons light mayonnaise; toss well. Serve with 1 whole wheat roll (about 80 calories). For dessert, have 1 fat-free Fudgsicle.

Day 15 Dinner. Mixed Greens with White Beans and Tuna

In a serving bowl, combine 2 cups mixed greens with 1 cup fresh broccoli florets and 1 chopped tomato. Add ½ cup rinsed and drained canned white beans, 3 ounces rinsed and drained chunk light water-packed tuna, ½ peeled and sectioned medium grapefruit, 1 tablespoon extra-virgin olive oil, 1 tablespoon rice vinegar, and 1 tablespoon capers; toss well. For dessert, have 3 meringue cookies.

Day 16 Dinner. "Fried Rice" with Tofu and Vegetables

In a medium skillet, heat 2 teaspoons sesame oil over medium heat. Add 2 ounces chopped firm tofu made with calcium sulfate, and cook, stirring occasionally, for 2 minutes. Add ⅔ cup cooked brown rice, ⅓ cup thawed frozen peas, ¼ cup grated carrots, 1 thinly sliced scallion, 1 tablespoon slivered almonds, 2 teaspoons reduced-sodium soy sauce, and ½ teaspoon minced garlic. Cook, stirring frequently, for 3 to 4 minutes, or until heated through. For dessert, have 1 cup fresh or canned (juice- or water-packed) pineapple.

Day 17 Dinner. White Fish with Baked Sweet Potato Fries

Preheat the oven to 350°F. Coat a baking dish with cooking spray. In a large zipper-lock bag, combine 2 tablespoons apricot preserves, 1 tablespoon lemon juice, 1 teaspoon extra-virgin olive oil, and ½ teaspoon cooking sherry. Add one (4-ounce) fillet of any white fish, such as tilapia or snapper, turn it to coat it, and marinate it in the refrigerator for 10 minutes. Cut one (4-ounce) sweet potato into ½"-thick "fries." Place them in the baking dish, drizzle them with 2 teaspoons extra-virgin olive oil, and sprinkle them with ½ teaspoon each paprika and black pepper. Bake for 15 minutes, then add the fish to the baking dish next to the potatoes and continue to bake for 15 minutes more, or until the fish is opaque and flakes easily with a fork. For dessert, have 1 frozen fruit juice bar (about 80 calories).

Day 18 Dinner. Fast Falafel

Prepare 1 serving of falafel, such as Fantastic Foods Falafel, according to the package directions, using ¼ cup dry mix and 2 teaspoons canola oil. In a serving bowl, combine 2 cups shredded romaine lettuce, ½ cup thinly sliced red bell pepper, and 1 sliced tomato. In a cup, combine ⅓ cup finely chopped cucumber, ⅓ cup plain low-fat yogurt, and 1 teaspoon minced garlic. Stuff the cooked falafel into one (6½") whole wheat pita and top with 3 tablespoons yogurt dressing. Top the salad with the remaining dressing and toss. For dessert, have 1 fat-free Fudgsicle.

Day 19 Dinner. Baked Acorn Squash with Whole Wheat Couscous

Preheat the oven to 375°F. Cut an acorn squash in half and remove the seeds. Place both halves cut side up in a baking dish, drizzle them with 2 teaspoons extra-virgin olive oil, and sprinkle them with ½ teaspoon each brown sugar and ground cinnamon. Bake for 50 minutes, or until the squash is softened. Meanwhile, prepare ½ cup cooked whole wheat couscous according to the package directions and toss with 1 chopped tomato, 1 minced clove garlic, and ¼ teaspoon dried basil; keep it warm. Serve the squash with the couscous. For dessert, have 1 sugar-free frozen fruit juice bar.

Day 20 Dinner. Quinoa Salad

In a medium saucepan, bring ½ cup water to a boil. Add ¼ cup dry quinoa, reduce the heat, and simmer, covered, for 9 minutes. Remove the pan from the heat and let the quinoa cool. For the dressing, in a cup, whisk together 2 tablespoons apple juice, 1 teaspoon honey, 1 teaspoon reduced-sodium soy sauce, ⅛ teaspoon curry powder, and a pinch of cayenne pepper. In a medium bowl, combine the quinoa with 1 finely chopped green bell pepper, 1 finely chopped medium apple, and 2 finely chopped celery stalks. Add the dressing and toss well. Top the salad with 1½ tablespoons chopped walnuts. For dessert, have 3 Hershey's Kisses.

Day 21 Dinner. Whole Wheat Pasta with Chickpeas

In a serving bowl, combine ½ cup rinsed and drained canned chickpeas, ½ cup cooked whole wheat pasta (any shape), 1 chopped tomato, 1 tablespoon Parmesan cheese, ½ teaspoon dried basil, 1 teaspoon minced garlic, and 1 teaspoon olive oil; toss well. For dessert, have 1 Skinny Cow Ice Cream Sandwich.

Day 22 Dinner. Teriyaki Swordfish with Romaine Salad

Preheat the oven to 350°F. Coat a baking dish with cooking spray. In a large zipper-lock bag, combine 1½ teaspoons reduced-sodium teriyaki sauce, 1 teaspoon sesame oil, ½ teaspoon minced garlic, and ½ teaspoon grated lemon peel. Add one (3-ounce) swordfish steak, turn it to coat it, and marinate it in the refrigerator for 10 minutes. Transfer the swordfish and marinade to the baking dish and bake for 15 minutes, or until the fish is opaque and flakes easily with a fork. For the salad, combine 1½ cups torn romaine lettuce leaves, 1 chopped small tomato, ¼ cup grated carrot, and 2 tablespoons light salad dressing of your choice (about 80 calories); toss well. Top with 3 tablespoons roasted soy nuts. For dessert, have 1 frozen fruit juice bar (about 80 calories).

Day 23 Dinner. Mushroom Beef and Bulgur Stroganoff

Coat a medium saucepan with cooking spray and heat over medium heat. Add 4 ounces round, sirloin, or flank steak cut into 1" pieces and cook, stirring occasionally, for 2 minutes, or until browned on all sides. Add ½ cup reduced-fat and reduced-sodium cream of mushroom soup (such as Campbell's Healthy Request), ½ cup chopped carrot, ½ cup sliced white mushrooms, ¼ cup dry bulgur, and ¼ cup water; stir well. Cover the pan tightly and cook for 8 minutes. Turn off the heat and let it sit, covered, for 15 minutes before serving. For dessert, have 1 frozen fruit juice bar (about 80 calories).

Day 24 Dinner. Minestrone Soup with Pita Triangles

Heat 2 cups of minestrone soup, such as Campbell's Healthy Request, and transfer it to a serving bowl. Top with 2 tablespoons shredded mozzarella cheese and half of a 6½" toasted whole wheat pita, cut into triangles. For dessert, have 1 Skinny Cow Ice Cream Sandwich.

Day 25 Dinner. Orange-Glazed Salmon and Broccoli with Almonds

Preheat the oven to 400°F. Coat a baking dish with cooking spray. Place one (4-ounce) salmon fillet in the baking dish and drizzle it with 1 tablespoon white wine and 1 teaspoon reduced-sodium soy sauce. Bake for 8 to 10 minutes, or until the fish is opaque and flakes easily with a fork. Meanwhile, steam 1 cup broccoli florets until crisp-tender; keep them warm. Coat a small saucepan with cooking spray and heat it over medium-high heat. Add ¼ cup calcium-fortified orange juice, 1 teaspoon cooking sherry, and ¼ teaspoon grated orange peel. Cook, stirring frequently, for 3 to 5 minutes, or until the sauce thickens. Transfer the salmon and broccoli to a serving plate, drizzle them with the sauce, and top them with 1 tablespoon slivered almonds. For dessert, have 1 cup frozen grapes.

Day 26 Dinner. A Southwest-Style Dinner (*Dine-Out Option*)

At Applebee's, order the Onion Soup au Gratin and the Cajun Lime Tilapia from the Weight Watchers menu. At T.G.I. Friday's, order a cup of French onion soup and the Santa Fe Chicken Salad (eat only half of the salad: split it with your dining partner or take some home). Elsewhere, order a cup of French onion soup and a Southwest-style chicken salad. Leave the cheese off the salad and portion out about 4 ounces chicken breast (the size of a bar of soap) and ½ cup each black beans, corn, peppers, and tomatoes. Ask for the light dressing of your choice on the side and use 2 tablespoons of it. For dessert, have 1 frozen fruit juice bar (about 80 calories) at home.

Day 27 Dinner. Mexican Soup

In a medium saucepan, combine 1 cup low-sodium chicken broth, 1 cup rinsed and drained canned kidney beans, ½ cup rinsed and drained canned black beans, 1 chopped tomato, 3 sliced baby carrots, ¼ cup chopped yellow or white onion, 1 chopped celery stalk, 1 tablespoon balsamic vinegar, and ½ teaspoon each chili powder and cumin. Stir well and bring to a boil over high heat. Reduce the heat to medium-low and simmer for 20 minutes, adding water during cooking, if needed. Transfer the soup to a serving bowl and top with 1 tablespoon Parmesan cheese. For dessert, have 3 meringue cookies.

Day 28 Dinner. Whole Wheat Couscous with Toasted Pine Nuts

Toast 1½ tablespoons pine nuts in a dry skillet over medium heat for 1 minute, stirring constantly; do not let them burn. In a serving bowl, combine 1 cup broccoli florets, ½ cup sliced orange bell pepper; ½ cup cooked whole wheat couscous, 1 tablespoon lemon juice, 1 teaspoon minced garlic, and 1 teaspoon olive oil; toss well. Top with the toasted pine nuts. For dessert, have 1 fat-free Fudgsicle.

Day 29 Dinner. Amy's Kitchen Indian Mattar Paneer

Heat 1 Amy's Kitchen Indian Mattar Paneer according to the package directions (or choose another frozen entrée with 320 calories and less than 8 grams saturated fat). For dessert, have 3 meringue cookies and 1 medium apple.

Day 30 Dinner. Scallop Stew

Prepare 1 cup cooked brown rice; keep it warm. While the rice is cooking, in a Dutch oven or covered casserole, combine one (8-ounce) can no-salt-added diced tomatoes (with liquid); 1 chopped green bell pepper; ¼ cup chopped onion; 1 minced clove garlic; ⅛ teaspoon each dried basil, thyme, black pepper, and paprika; and a pinch of cayenne pepper; stir well. Cover the pan and cook over low heat for 20 minutes. Increase the heat to high and bring the stew to a boil. Add 4 ounces sea scallops and cook for 3 to 4 minutes, or until the scallops are just opaque. Serve immediately over the brown rice. For dessert, have 1 frozen fruit juice bar (about 80 calories).

Satisfying Snacks

Each of the snacks in the Natural Fat-Loss Pharmacy Meal Plan provides about 250 calories. Repeat your favorite snacks as often as you'd like. There are many easy-to-take-along options, so you can stick with your weight-loss plan no matter what's on your daily schedule.

Have your snack at any time of the day—but consider saving it for when you're especially hungry. Midmorning and midafternoon are likely times, as you well know. And, as you'll see, we've designed the plan so that some snacks are more congenial for the A.M. and some for the P.M.

Day 1 Snack. All-Bran Cereal Bar and Yogurt with Almonds

Have half of a Kellogg's All-Bran cereal bar, any flavor, with 1 cup plain low-fat yogurt topped with 1 tablespoon slivered almonds. Save the other half of the breakfast bar in a small zipper-lock bag and eat it for the Day 10 snack (page 298).

Day 2 Snack. Pria Bar and Milk

Have 1 Pria bar, any flavor, with 1 cup fat-free milk and 1 cup raspberries.

Day 3 Snack. Cereal, Yogurt, and Nuts

Have ¼ cup Kashi Good Friends cereal or Cheerios (or 30 calories' worth of another cereal with at least 3 grams fiber per 1 cup serving) sprinkled over 1 cup plain low-fat yogurt. Top with 1½ tablespoons chopped walnuts.

Day 4 Snack. Smoothie of Your Choice

Have 1 Yoplait Nouriche SuperSmoothie or any prepared smoothie with at least 300 mg calcium and about 260 calories.

Day 5 Snack. Blueberry Muffin

Have 1 Weight Watchers fat-free Blueberry Muffin (or any 170-calorie muffin) and 1 cup light chocolate soy milk.

Day 6 Snack. Fruit and Cheese Wrap

Top 1 whole wheat soft tortilla (such as a Flatout Healthy Grains wrap or a soft tortilla with 140 calories and at least 4 grams fiber) with 2 slices soy cheese, such as Veggie Slices (or any soy cheese with 35 calories and 200 mg calcium per slice), and 1 tablespoon raisins; roll it up.

Day 7 Snack. Peanut Butter and Apricot Crackers

Spread 1 slice Wasa brand cracker or 2 small whole wheat crackers (look for 40 calories and at least 1 gram fiber per serving) with 1 tablespoon peanut butter. Top with 2 dried apricot halves and serve with 1½ cups light vanilla soy milk for drinking.

Day 8 Snack. Almond Butter Waffle

Toast 1 whole grain waffle, such as Kashi GOLEAN Original. Top with 2 teaspoons almond butter or peanut butter. Serve with 1 cup light chocolate soy milk for drinking.

Day 9 Snack. Hearty Honey Oatmeal

In a serving bowl, combine ¼ cup low-fat ricotta cheese with 1 teaspoon brown sugar and 1 teaspoon honey. Make 1 packet unflavored instant oatmeal or ½ cup regular oatmeal according to the package directions, using ½ cup fat-free milk. Stir the oatmeal into the ricotta cheese mixture.

Day 10 Snack. All-Bran Cereal Bar and Yogurt with Walnuts

Have half of a Kellogg's All-Bran cereal bar, any flavor, with 1 cup plain low-fat yogurt. Top with 1 tablespoon chopped walnuts.

Day 11 Snack. Cheesy Cinnamon Toast

Preheat the oven to 200°F. Top 1 slice whole wheat bread, such as Healthy Choice Hearty 100% Whole Grain, with 1 slice veggie cheese (such as Veggie Slices or any soy cheese with 35 calories and 200 mg calcium per slice). Sprinkle with ½ teaspoon brown sugar and a pinch of ground cinnamon. Toast it in the oven until the cheese is melted, about 2 minutes. Serve it with ¾ cup strawberries and 1 cup light chocolate soy milk for drinking.

Day 12 Snack. Blackberry Oatmeal

Make 1 packet unflavored instant oatmeal or ½ cup regular oatmeal according to the package directions, using ½ cup fat-free milk. Top with ½ cup fresh or frozen unsweetened blackberries, ½ teaspoon brown sugar, and ⅛ teaspoon ground cinnamon. Serve with 1 cup fat-free milk to drink.

Day 13 Snack. Soy Nuts and Café au Lait

Have ¼ cup soy nuts along with café au lait made with 1½ cups fat-free milk mixed with 1½ cups brewed coffee and 2 teaspoons sweetened coffee creamer.

Day 14 Snack. Popcorn with Apple and Cheese

Pop a bag of 94% reduced-fat microwaveable popcorn according to the package directions. Have 4 cups popcorn along with 1 sliced medium apple topped with 2 slices soy cheese (such as Veggie Slices or any soy cheese with 35 calories and 200 mg calcium per slice).

Day 15 Snack. Ricotta–Peanut Butter Spread with Graham Crackers
Mix ½ cup low-fat ricotta cheese with 1 tablespoon peanut butter and 1 teaspoon brown sugar. Eat with 2 plain graham cracker squares (1 sheet graham crackers) for dipping.

Day 16 Snack. Waffle with Fruit and Milk
Toast 1 whole grain waffle (such as Kashi GOLEAN Original) and top with ½ cup blueberries. Serve with 2 cups light vanilla soy milk for drinking.

Day 17 Snack. Pump 'n' Cheese
Preheat the oven to 200°F. Top 1 slice pumpernickel bread with 1 slice soy cheese and heat in the oven for 2 to 3 minutes, or until the cheese is slightly melted. Serve with 1 orange and 1 cup fat-free milk for drinking.

Day 18 Snack. Apricot Cottage Cheese
Mix ½ cup 1% or fat-free cottage cheese with 2 teaspoons apricot jam and ¼ teaspoon vanilla extract. Serve with 2 cups light vanilla soy milk for drinking.

Day 19 Snack. Cheese Nachos
Place about 9 baked tortilla chips (0.5 ounce) on a microwaveable plate. Top with 2 slices 2% American or Cheddar cheese, broken into small pieces. Heat in a microwave oven on high power for 60 to 90 seconds, or until the cheese begins to melt. Top with 4 tablespoons salsa.

Day 20 Snack. Crunchy Fruity Yogurt Bowl
Top ¼ cup low-fat granola cereal, such as Kellogg's or Healthy Choice, with 1 cup plain low-fat yogurt and 1 chopped medium peach or 2 chopped medium plums.

Day 21 Snack. Veggies with Onion Dip
Coat a medium skillet with cooking spray and heat over medium heat. Add ½ cup chopped onion and 1 finely chopped shallot. Cook, stirring

occasionally, for 3 to 4 minutes, or until translucent. Add 1 teaspoon minced garlic and stir for 1 minute more; remove the pan from the heat and transfer the contents to a medium bowl. Add ⅔ cup low-fat sour cream, 2 teaspoons light canola oil mayonnaise, and a pinch of cayenne pepper (the dip will be chunky). Divide the dip in half. Serve one half with 10 baby carrots and 10 cherry tomatoes for dipping and 1 cup fat-free soy milk for drinking. Save the other half of the dip in the refrigerator for the Day 23 snack or for up to 3 days.

Day 22 Snack. Crackers with Tahini
Spread 1 slice Wasa brand cracker or 3 reduced-fat Triscuit crackers (or 100 calories' worth of your favorite whole wheat, trans-fat-free cracker) with 1 tablespoon tahini. Serve with ¾ cup strawberries and 1½ cups light vanilla soy milk for drinking.

Day 23 Snack. Broccoli with Onion Dip
Serve the reserved half of the Onion Dip from the Day 21 snack with 1½ cups uncooked broccoli florets for dipping.

Day 24 Snack. Creamy Raspberry Smoothie
In a blender, combine 1 cup fresh or frozen unsweetened raspberries (if using frozen berries, don't thaw them for a really thick, frosty smoothie), 6 ounces plain low-fat yogurt, 5 tablespoons calcium-fortified orange juice, 2 ounces tofu made with calcium sulfate, and ¼ teaspoon vanilla extract. Blend until smooth.

Day 25 Snack. Fruit Bowl with Cheddar and Milk
Combine 1 cup blueberries and 1 sliced kiwifruit. Serve with 1 slice 2% American or Cheddar cheese and 1 cup fat-free milk for drinking.

Day 26 Snack. Maple Graham Crackers
Mix ⅓ cup low-fat ricotta cheese with 1½ tablespoons maple syrup. Serve with 3 plain graham cracker squares for dipping.

300-CALORIE SUPER SNACKS

These snacks aren't for everybody. So who *should* eat them? You should . . . if you have been on the plan for a week or so—including eating your daily 250-calorie snack—and find you're still hungry; if you exercise five or more days a week, for at least one hour; or if you've reached your goal weight.

Also, some larger men—guys who can eat more than 1,500 calories a day and still lose weight—may also want to eat one of these 300-calorie snacks in addition to the 250-calorie snack.

In other words, you can eat breakfast, lunch, dinner, the 250-calorie snack, *and* one of the 300-calorie snacks below.

- 1 fat-free Yoplait Nouriche SuperSmoothie (any flavor)

- 1 cup Kashi Heart to Heart cereal with ¾ cup fat-free milk and a 1-ounce stick string cheese

- 1 banana spread with 2 tablespoons peanut butter

- 1 Clif bar (any flavor) with 1 small apple

- 1 cup fruit-flavored low-fat yogurt with 2 tablespoons raisins

- 2 hard taco shells (check the label for 0 grams trans fats and no partially hydrogenated oils in the ingredients) filled with ¼ cup rinsed and drained canned kidney beans and 1 tablespoon shredded Cheddar cheese. Heat in a microwave oven on high power for 1 minute.

- 1 whole wheat soft tortilla (such as a Flatout brand Healthy Grains wrap or a soft tortilla with 140 calories and at least 4 grams fiber) spread with 2 tablespoons light cream cheese and topped with 3 tablespoons Craisins cherry flavor sweetened dried cranberries

- 2 cups chicken noodle soup, such as Healthy Choice brand, with 10 reduced-fat Wheat Thins crackers

- 12-ounce fat-free latte with 1 plain (undipped) biscotti and 2 tablespoons mixed nuts

- One (6½") whole wheat pita filled with egg salad made from 1 large hard-cooked egg mixed with 1 tablespoon light canola oil mayonnaise

Day 27 Snack. English Muffin with Peanut Butter and Soy Milk
Spread half of a toasted whole wheat English muffin with 2 teaspoons peanut butter. Serve with 1½ cups light chocolate soy milk for drinking.

Day 28 Snack. Two-Berry Smoothie
In a blender, combine 1 cup fresh or frozen unsweetened blackberries and ½ cup fresh or frozen unsweetened strawberries (if using frozen berries, don't thaw them for a really thick, frosty smoothie), 1 cup fat-free milk, 2 ounces tofu made with calcium sulfate, 1 tablespoon wheat germ, and ¼ teaspoon almond or vanilla extract. Blend until smooth.

Day 29 Snack. Blueberry Muffin with a Latte
Have half a Weight Watchers fat-free Blueberry Muffin with a 16-ounce fat-free latte.

Day 30 Snack. Pear with Peanut Butter and Yogurt
Spread 1 sliced small pear with 1 teaspoon peanut butter. Serve with 1 cup plain low-fat yogurt.

LOW CALORIE DENSITY: HOW TO EAT A LOT AND LOSE WEIGHT

Now, for another way to lose weight, let's go to Florida, where people are shedding pounds by eating all they want, six times a day. "We know the bottom line in weight loss is 'calories in versus calories out,'" says Jeffrey Novick, MS, RD, director of nutrition at the Pritikin Longevity Center in Aventura, Florida. But something happened to those calories on the way to the supermarket. Oranges turned into orange soda. Corn into corn chips. And chicken into chicken nuggets.

"In the last thirty to forty years, the food industry has figured out new ways to process and refine foods that *concentrate* calories," Novick told us.

For instance, let's compare two 100-calorie snacks: 2¾ cups of strawberries and . . . ten jellybeans. Both deliver the same number of calories. But

100 calories of jellybeans is a tiny portion, while 100 calories of strawberries is practically a meal. That's because jellybeans have an extremely high *calorie density*.

And if you're a jellybean fan, it's easy to imagine eating twenty or more of them in a couple of minutes. (I'll have a cherry and a licorice and a cinnamon and a coconut . . .) You probably couldn't even finish eating their caloric equivalent in strawberries: 5½ cups!

You're probably getting the calorie density picture.

Foods *high* in calorie density—baked goods like crackers and bagels; sweets like cookies; nuts and seeds; fats like butter and oils—are *easy* to overeat.

Foods *low* in calorie density—fruits; vegetables; and what Novick calls "unrefined, naturally occurring complex carbohydrates" like potatoes (not French-fried), rice, peas, and corn—are *hard* to overeat. They're packed with fiber and water, filling you up and satisfying your hunger, so that you don't need or want to keep eating (what nutritionists dub *satiety*). In fact, with low-calorie-density foods, you can eat *all you want*, and still not overdo it on calories.

40 Percent More Weight Loss—On Low-Calorie-Density Foods

In a study conducted by one of the top experts on calorie density and satiety—Barbara Rolls, PhD, a professor of nutrition at Pennsylvania State University—two hundred overweight and obese men and women went on the same low-calorie diet for one year.

One group, however, ate one serving a day of soup that was low in calorie density. Another group ate two servings a day of the soup. A third group ate two servings a day of calorie-dense snack food. At the end of the year, which group lost the most weight?

The two-soup-a-day group lost an average of 17.8 pounds. The one-soup-a-day group lost 13.4 pounds. The snack group lost 10.6 pounds.

"Consuming foods that are low in energy [calorie] density can be an effective strategy for weight management," concluded Dr. Rolls and her colleagues in the June 2005 issue of *Obesity Research*.

A Guide to Calorie Density

Novick says the best way to think about calorie density is to think of foods in terms of *calories per pound*. Sure, you wouldn't eat a pound of broccoli or a pound of butter. But a pound-for-pound comparison between the two foods shows just how many calories each packs and the differences between them.

100 to 200 calories per pound. In this range are the vegetables, with leafy greens the lowest in calorie density.

200 to 300 calories per pound. These are the fresh fruits, like oranges and berries. Bananas are a little higher, at around 400, but still very low on the overall scale, as you'll see in a moment.

500 calories per pound. These are (as we mentioned earlier) what Novick calls the "unrefined, naturally occurring complex carbohydrates," like potatoes, rice, peas, and corn.

600 to 650 calories per pound. This category includes lean proteins, like seafood and the white meat of chicken. Beans are also in this range.

1,000 calories per pound. Here you'll find the fatty proteins, like the steaks served at restaurants that specialize in "premium" steaks. You'll also find whole wheat varieties of pasta, tortillas, pitas, wraps, bread, and bagels.

1,200 to 1,500 calories per pound. These are what Novick calls the "refined, processed carbohydrates," like white-flour breads, bagels, and crackers. Whole wheat crackers also fall into this category, but they're a healthy food when eaten in moderation—which is just how they're featured in the Natural Fat-Loss Pharmacy Meal Plan.

2,000 calories per pound. Now we're in the land of "junk food," says Novick, like super-sugary cookies made with white flour.

2,800 calories per pound. Nuts and seeds comprise this category.

4,000 calories per pound. These are the oils and fats, like butter.

For Weight Loss, Stay at 600 and Below

"If you eat foods that are 600 calories per pound and less, and you're fairly active (thirty minutes of exercise most days of the week), you can eat as much as you want and still lose weight," says Novick. And, he points out, you won't have to count calories or measure portions.

If you eat in the 650 to 1,000 range and you're fairly active, you'll probably maintain weight. If you're not active, you're likely to gain.

When the majority of your foods are 1,000 calories per pound or higher—you'll probably gain weight.

People attending the Pritikin Longevity Institute are treated to an unlimited buffet of foods in the 400 or lower range, six times a day: breakfast, lunch, dinner, two snacks, and a "happy hour." But that doesn't mean they're only eating fruits and vegetables. They also eat unrefined carbohydrates and lean meats, using a trick Novick calls *dilution*.

Dilute Higher-Density Foods

"Pasta, for example, is around 500 calories per pound," says Novick. "But if you dilute it with vegetables—if you make pasta primavera with half pasta and half vegetables—you dramatically reduce the calorie density." Do the same with lean protein, mixing it with vegetables in salads and stir-fry.

Burn Fat Instead of Muscle

This way of eating has advantages beyond cutting calories, says Dr. Preuss. It also cuts way (way) down on refined carbohydrates. A diet lower in calories *and* refined carbs doesn't inundate your insulin system, which regulates blood sugar. The result: your body tends to burn *fat* instead of muscle. (As we explained at length in several other chapters, loss of *muscle* during dieting is one reason why so many people regain weight.)

The diet Novick recommends also doesn't eliminate lean protein, as some low-fat and vegetarian approaches advise. Protein helps boost metabolic rate by up to 30 percent, burning more calories, says Dr. Preuss. It also sparks the system to release the hormone *glucagon*, which pries stored fat out of tissues, so it can be burned up.

Another advantage of this approach, says Dr. Preuss, is that it completely eliminates *trans fats*—the so-called *partially hydrogenated* fats found primarily in baked goods and the deep-fried foods served in restaurants, from French fries to chicken to fish. Many experts say trans fats are coronary transgressors: they invade arteries and increase the risk of heart attacks. Saying good riddance is a good idea.

But if you want to be metabolically merry, you have to pay attention to what you eat *and* drink, says Dr. Preuss. Choose no-calorie-density water over soft drinks, fruit juices, and full-fat milk. Drink at least six 8-ounce glasses of water a day. And speaking of soda . . .

Caution: Huge Portions Ahead!

If you're a boomer or older, you probably remember when sodas came in 6-ounce bottles. Now, 32 ounces (or more) is a "normal" serving. Portions have become preposterous. And many studies by Dr. Rolls and her colleagues prove the obvious: when you present people with bigger portions of calorie-dense food, they eat a whole lot more calories.

"And the bigger the plate or serving," says Novick, "the more you're likely to eat." That's good news when you go to the salad bar—take a bigger plate! But otherwise be on the alert in restaurants, he says. "When you're given a huge plate of food, don't eat it all."

The Downside of Variety

Novick also points out that if you're offered many *types* of foods at a single meal, you're more likely to overdo it on calories. When you eat in the 400-calorie-per-pound or under range, you *should* emphasize variety: eat lots of different vegetables and fruits. Aside from fruits and vegetables, however, simpler is smarter.

"When you sit down at your dinner table, have a piece of chicken and a starch and a vegetable," he says. "Don't have two starches and two types of protein."

The 90 Percent Solution

Don't worry if you don't stay below 600 calories per pound 100 percent of the time. "Obviously, you're going to eat some foods that are calorie dense," says Novick. "But try to keep 90 percent of your intake in the lower range. Get *most* of what you eat right."

THE CALORIE BUDGET

The Natural Fat-Loss Pharmacy Meal Plan will help you lose weight. But some people don't like a plan—and maybe you're one of them. Maybe you'd rather figure out the amount of calories you need to lose weight and then eat whatever you want within that range. If that's your preference, don't worry. We've got help for you.

We talked with Susan Luke, RD, registered dietician, nutrition counselor, and president of trEAT WELL Nutrition Services in Charlotte, North Carolina. She specializes in weight loss and sports nutrition. Her clients include the 2008 Olympic kayaking and canoeing teams and the Bobcats of the NBA, and she has served as the nutritionist for the NBA's Charlotte

Hornets, the WNBA's Charlotte Sting, and for Disney on Ice. "To me, the bottom line in weight management is calories, just like the bottom line in money management is dollars," she says.

"How can you manage your money if you don't know the value of dollars?" she asks. "Similarly, how can you manage your weight if you don't know where calories are found?"

Luke works with her clients to create a *calorie budget*. "Most of us understand the concept of budgeting," she told us. "You have a certain amount of money and you have to find creative ways to stay within your budget—to not overspend. Just so, you have a certain number of calories you can eat every day without gaining weight, and you have to find ways to not eat more than that amount." Here's how she helps her clients do just that.

Figure Out What You *Can* Spend

Once you know how many calories you need to maintain your weight, your next step is learning to keep track of your daily intake. It's not hard, says Luke.

An easy way to estimate your daily need for calories, says Luke, is at the Web site www.mypyramid.gov, the USDA guide to the food pyramid. On the home page, under "My Pyramid Plan," enter your gender, age, and daily activity level. The site will then give you a *calorie pattern*. For example, a forty-year-old woman who exercises thirty minutes a day needs 2,000 calories to maintain her weight, while an inactive sixty-year-old man needs 2,200. A commercial site where you can calculate your daily calories with a little more accuracy is www.caloriecontrol.org: use the "Weight Maintenance Calculator" on the home page.

Figure Out What You *Do* Spend

Once you know how many calories you need to maintain your weight, your next step is learning to keep track of your daily intake. It's not hard, says Novick.

Keep a food diary. Carry a small notebook or a few index cards with you, and jot down the foods you eat. At the end of the day, look up their calorie count.

Buy the best book. Luke recommends *The Complete Book of Food Counts* by Corinne T. Netzer. She finds it easy to use because it's organized alphabetically (rather than by food group), updated frequently, and includes fast foods (which just about everybody eats now and then).

It's easier than you think—because you won't be tracking a lot of foods. "Most people eat about four different breakfasts, four or five lunches, and ten dinners," Luke told us. "And at those meals, they tend to eat the same ten or fifteen foods over and over again. It doesn't take very long to figure out the calories of the foods you're choosing to eat every day, because you don't eat that many different foods."

Spend 250 Calories a Day Less

Luke instructs her clients to think about their calorie budgets—and how they're going to spend 250 calories a day less. (To burn extra calories, she also advises her clients to take up *joyful movement*—any activity, from walking to belly dancing, that they truly enjoy.)

That level of calorie reduction will accomplish a weight loss of half a pound per week. And that's the best pace for *permanent* weight loss. "The slower the weight comes off, the more likely it is that you'll never see it again," says Luke.

Here are some of her other tips for a lifetime of healthy eating, weight loss and maintenance, and easy calorie control.

Prioritize pleasure. The most important principle for a lifetime of healthy eating is *taste*, says Luke. "If your food choices don't taste good to you, you're not going to stick with them."

Turn your plate into a peace symbol. Imagine a peace symbol, she says. Now pretend it is your plate. The bottom, or smallest area, should contain lean protein, like fish or chicken. One of the two upper, larger areas should contain starch, with the emphasis on complex carbohydrates. The other upper area should contain vegetables.

Don't let yourself get too hungry. If you're not *too* hungry when you eat, you'll make rational, intelligent choices. If you're ravenous, however, you'll tend to overeat. Never go longer than five hours without eating, says Luke.

Save a little bit of the budget "just for me." About three-fourths of your budget should consist of good, balanced food choices, like those on the "peace symbol plate." Spend the remaining fourth in whatever way you like. "Say I have $20 to spend," says Luke. "I keep $15 in one pocket for necessities. In the other pocket is $5—and that's 'just for me.' "

Don't get obsessed. Finally, says Luke, you should be easygoing about calorie control. "There's no need to obsessively count calories. Learn the concept of calorie budgeting—and then be loose about it. It should fit you like a comfortable pair of bedroom slippers."

Self-love: The Opposite of Overeating

But overeating isn't all about calories, says Luke. A common cause of overeating is a *lack of self-love*. "A lot of people are walking around feeling empty," she told us. "They turn to food to fill up a hungry heart. It doesn't work. But they keep trying."

There are two clues that reveal you may be what Luke calls an "emotional eater": eating when you're not hungry; and continuing to eat when you're full.

Another is choosing food you know isn't good for you. "Food is nourishment," says Luke. "Food is health. Food is gasoline for our bodies. If you're choosing to put cheap gasoline in your tank, what is that about? Do you feel that is all you deserve?"

She counsels clients who may be emotional eaters to talk to a therapist—a professional who can help them uncover and understand what their relationship to food signifies on an emotional level.

She also has some practical tips for emotional eaters and anyone who wants to eat with love:

Eat slowly and savor what you're eating. You deserve to taste what you're eating—and not wolf it down before anybody sees you.

Eat in full view of others. This helps you avoid "shameful eating," says Luke.

Eat what you want to eat, not what you think you should eat. Make food choices based on self-love—because you deserve to be healthy and have good energy, and not because you'll be "bad" if you eat certain foods.

Designate a spot for eating. Eating in front of the TV or in the car is not about self-love. Pick a comfortable spot, sit down, relax, and *enjoy* what you're eating.

Treat yourself with respect. "Most people take better care of their cars than their bodies," says Luke. "But you can trade in your car. This is the only body you're ever going to get. Treat it with respect, and feed it with love."

DO YOU NEED A NUTRITIONAL SUPPLEMENT?

Luke advises her clients—particularly those who say they hate vegetables—to take a daily multivitamin-mineral supplement. "I recommend they purchase any reliable, inexpensive brand." Should a supplement be part of *your* nutritional strategy?

To find out, we talked with Heather Pena, MD, Medical Director of the St. Helena Center for Health, at the St. Helena Hospital in California's Napa Valley. Dr. Pena supervises Transformations: The Napa Valley Weight and Lifestyle Management Program, where every participant receives a customized recommendation about nutritional supplements. Here's her advice on figuring out if you need a supplement or not.

You probably don't need a supplement if . . .

You get more than five servings a day of fruits and vegetables, plenty of fiber, and healthy fats (like those found in fish, avocado, and olive oil) in reasonable amounts.

But most people *don't* eat like that, says Dr. Pena. "Except for those with a remarkable knowledge and practice of nutrition, most people will benefit from a good multivitamin-mineral supplement," she says.

You probably do need a supplement if . . .

And depending on what you eat and the medications you take, you may be at extra risk for nutritional deficits, says Dr. Pena. For example:

You eat a lot of refined carbohydrates. Sugar and white flour can steal B vitamins from your body.

You don't get much sun. Exposure to sunlight is the only way your body makes vitamin D. And you're particularly at risk for low levels if you don't drink milk, one of the few foods fortified with the nutrient.

You take a diuretic. This class of drug—often prescribed for high blood pressure—is known to drain the body of potassium, and doctors may prescribe a potassium supplement with a diuretic. But diuretics can also steal vitamin B$_1$ and the mineral magnesium.

You take an antacid. "Over time, acid-blocking drugs can rob the body of vitamin B$_{12}$," says Dr. Pena.

You're on a low-calorie diet. Low-calorie diets can cause suboptimal intake of many nutrients, she says, including B vitamins and calcium.

You're diabetic. "Diabetics don't make or utilize beta-carotene very well, and need it in a supplement," says Dr. Pena.

You don't eat fatty fish like salmon. Along with a multiple, Dr. Pena often recommends a fish oil supplement, which contains omega-3 fatty acids. "This type of fat is anti-inflammatory, protects the heart, and strengthens brain cells," she says. "If you eat fatty fish like salmon twice a week, you don't have to take this supplement. Otherwise, it's a good idea."

Other doctors agree with Dr. Pena about omega-3 fatty acids. In fact, some think it's the number one food supplement for better health.

OMEGA-3: THE ESSENTIAL FAT

"I put every patient I see on a supplement of omega-3 essential fatty acids," says Leigh Erin Connealy, MD. "It is the most important supplement a person can take."

There are two kinds of omega-3 supplements: fish oil supplements, rich in DHA (docosahexaenoic acid) and EPA (eicosahexaenoic acid), and plant-derived supplements, rich in ALA (alpha-linoleic acid), a fatty acid that converts to DHA and EPA in the body.

Why does Dr. Connealy favor these supplements? Omega-3 fatty acids strengthen the cell membrane, or outer covering. This aids in cell-to-cell communication, a crucial process in health. Omega-3 also decreases inflammation, which is linked to many different diseases, including heart disease, cancer, arthritis, and Alzheimer's. Omega-3 plays a role in *every* physiological function in the body, says Dr. Connealy.

Hundreds of scientific studies on omega-3 fatty acids show they can strengthen the heart, boost emotional well-being, improve memory and learning, and decrease joint pain. Let's look at some recent research . . .

Heart Disease

Heart attack. In a study conducted by Italian researchers, more than eleven thousand people who had suffered a heart attack took an omega-3 supplement or underwent another type of medical, dietary, or nutritional therapy. Among those who took omega-3, there were 30 percent fewer deaths and 20 percent fewer second heart attacks (*Journal of Membrane Biology*, 2005).

Sudden cardiac death. The study described above also reported 45 percent fewer cases of *cardiac arrhythmia*—an electrical abnormality in the heart (either *ventricular tachycardia* or *fibrillation*) that causes sudden cardiac death. (A heart attack is caused by a blockage in an artery to the heart.) Researchers at Harvard Medical School gave a supplement of either fish oil or olive oil to 402 heart patients with pacemakers, which help regulate the heart's electrical currents. After eleven months, those who took fish oil had a 38 percent lower death rate (*Circulation*, 2005).

Bypass surgery. Heart patients who took omega-3 fatty acids for five days before coronary bypass surgery had 55 percent fewer incidents of postoperative arterial fibrillation and shorter hospital stays than those who didn't take the supplement (*Journal of the American College of Cardiology*, 2005).

Inflammation

Arthritis. Neurosurgeons at the University of Pittsburgh gave fish oil supplements to 120 arthritis patients with neck or back pain. After seventy-five days, 68 percent of the patients had stopped taking prescription pain medications (*Surgical Neurology*, 2006).

Asthma. Sixteen asthmatic patients with exercise-induced bronchoconstriction (EIB)—an asthma attack brought on by exercise—were given either fish oil supplements or a placebo for six weeks. Those who took the supplement had reductions in many signs of inflammation (biochemicals called *interleukin, leukotriene,* and *cytokine*) and took less asthma medication (*Chest*, 2006).

Chronic obstructive pulmonary disease (COPD). Chronic lung disease (the fifth leading cause of death worldwide) is always accompanied by chronic inflammation. For two years, Japanese researchers gave sixty-four patients with COPD either a supplement rich in omega-3 or another treatment. Those taking omega-3 walked with less difficulty and had fewer signs of inflammation. "We suggest nutritional support with omega-3 . . . as a safe and practical method for treating COPD," concluded the researchers (*Chest*, 2005).

Alzheimer's disease. The brain changes of Alzheimer's disease involve inflammation. Researchers in the Veterans Affairs Healthcare System in Los Angeles had studied NSAIDs (nonsteroidal anti-inflammatory drugs, such as ibuprofen) as a treatment for the disease. Recent safety concerns about chronic use of NSAIDs led them to focus on natural anti-inflammatory treatments, like DHA. In studies on rats genetically altered to develop Alzheimer-like symptoms, DHA reduced the number of beta-amyloid plaques (found in the brain of Alzheimer's patients), decreased brain injury from free-radical molecules, improved transmission between brain cells, and boosted mental ability (*Neurobiology of Aging*, 2005).

DIET DÉCOR

No, we're not talking about slim sofas or trim tables. We're talking about "designing" your home and work environments so they match your goal of losing weight.

"You need to make sure your refrigerator, freezer, and shelves are stocked with foods conducive to your intention to get or stay trim," says Joan Salge Blake, MS, RD, a clinical assistant professor of nutrition at Boston University, author of *Nutrition and You*, and a weight-loss counselor in private practice. A few of her tips:

Stock the freezer with frozen vegetables. "Even if you haven't been able to go shopping for a couple of days because of your busy lifestyle, you'll be able to have plenty of vegetables on your plate at dinner," she told us.

Don't turn your home into a bakery. Stock a limited amount of sweets like low-fat ice cream, cookies, or candy, says Blake. "Those treats shouldn't be forbidden, but they also shouldn't be unlimited."

Bring a week's worth of snacks to work. "It's 3:30 P.M. and you're hungry—and you want filling, low-calorie fruits, vegetables, and low-fat dairy to be readily accessible," says Blake. Her solution? "Bring a crate of clementines to work, along with five containers of yogurt," says Blake. "You'll have an automatic, planned snack for every day of the week."

Lupus. Fifty-two patients with lupus (systemic lupus erythematosus, or SLE, a chronic autoimmune disease that can cause inflammation throughout the body) were given either fish oil supplements or a placebo. There was a significant decline in symptoms among those taking fish oil, compared to the placebo (*Journal of Rheumatology*, 2004).

Psychological Problems

Test anxiety. Students who received a supplement including omega-3 fatty acids had less test anxiety than students not getting the supplement (they were less nervous, slept better, concentrated better, had less fatigue, were more organized, and felt happier) (*Nutritional Neuroscience*, 2005).

Manic depression. People with manic depression (bipolar disorder) were given either EPA supplements or a placebo for several weeks. Those who took EPA had significantly less depression and mania. EPA, wrote the researchers, "is an effective and well-tolerated intervention in bipolar depression" (*British Journal of Psychiatry*, 2006).

Depression in diabetes. Depression is a common complication of type 2 diabetes, but antidepressant drugs only work in 50 to 60 percent of diabetic patients. Scientists in the Netherlands reviewed all the research on omega-3 supplements and depression in diabetics and concluded the supplement is a "safe and helpful tool to reduce the incidence of depression and to treat depression in Type 2 diabetes" (*Diabetic Medicine*, 2005).

Attention deficit hyperactivity disorder (ADHD). Researchers in India gave ALA supplements to children with ADHD, leading to a significant improvement in their symptoms (*Prostaglandins Leukotrienes and Essential Fatty Acids*, 2006).

What to Take

Throughout this book, we have recommended brands of supplements used in research studies that produced a positive result—because that's the brand scientific research indicates has the highest likelihood of actually working when you take it. For omega-3, we're recommending Nordic Naturals, the brand most widely used in scientific studies, including several of those reported in this section. Currently, Nordic Naturals is being tested at Duke University (for anxiety), the University of California, Davis (for exercise tolerance), Texas A&M University (for glucose tolerance),

Oregon Health Sciences University (for Alzheimer's disease), Cedars-Sinai Medical Center in New York (for depression), and at many other universities, hospitals, and research institutions. Nordic Naturals offers several different types of omega-3 products. Follow the dosage recommendation on the label.

Step Right Up to Weight Control

Use a Pedometer to Walk More— And Keep Off the Weight You've Lost

Right on Reservoir Road to 38th street (300 steps) . . . left on 38th to T Street (600 steps) . . . right on T to 35th (700 steps), down 35th to Volta Place (1,200 steps), left on Volta, for a stroll around the Georgetown Playground (400 steps) . . . and back to Georgetown University Medical Center.

That's Dr. Preuss, taking one of his postlunch walks around Georgetown, in the District of Columbia . . . accompanied by his trusty pedometer.

A pedometer is a small device that clips to your belt or waistband. It counts and displays the number of *steps* you take each day. And when it comes to pedometers, Dr. Preuss is a poster adult.

Every day, without fail, he puts on his pedometer—and walks 15,000 steps (an ambitious amount of daily walking that one study on pedometers describes as "highly active"). If he doesn't reach his goal—maybe because he's spent all day in an airplane flying to a scientific conference—he tries hard to "make up" his missed steps the next day. But Dr. Preuss isn't the only scientist passionate about pedometers.

At universities across the country, researchers are conducting study after study on walking programs using "step-count feedback" from a pedometer. And their research shows that putting on a pedometer may be one of the best ways to *not* regain the weight you've lost. Interested? If you're like tens of millions of Americans who've lost weight only to see the pounds creep back . . . if you've been a prisoner for years inside that vicious circle . . . you might be *very* interested. So step this way: we'll tell you everything you need to know about pedometers, steps, walking, and *permanent* weight loss.

REGULAR EXERCISE: THE BEST WAY TO KEEP WEIGHT OFF

Let's start with a surprising scientific fact: exercise is not the best way to *lose* weight. But it is the best way to not *gain* (or regain) weight. Case in point . . .

"Crucial in Successful Maintenance of Weight Loss"

Researchers from Duke University Medical Center reviewed all the "available evidence" on exercise and weight loss, publishing their results in the *American Heart Journal* in March 2006.

"Exercise alone is a relatively inefficient means for losing weight," they concluded. But, they continued, "regular exercise appears crucial in the *prevention* of weight gain and successful *maintenance* of weight loss." (Emphasis ours.)

Why is exercise effective for keeping weight off but not for taking it off?

To find out, we talked with James Hill, PhD, a professor at the University of Colorado, and coauthor of *The Step Diet*, which features pedometer-measured walking as an ideal way to help maintain weight.

Calorie Cutting and Calorie Burning

"It's simply a matter of math," he told us. "You can reduce your energy intake by 1,000 calories tomorrow. But if you're overweight and out of shape, you won't be able to burn 1,000 calories with exercise—in fact, you'll be lucky to burn an extra 100 calories." (It takes about thirty minutes of walking to burn 100 calories.)

"Exercise has an important but *secondary* role to play in losing weight," says Dr. Hill. "But to keep weight off—to stay at a normal weight or prevent weight regain—calorie restriction becomes secondary, and physical activity becomes the *absolute key* to success. And walking is the best way to stay active."

Walking: For Many, the Secret of Long-Term Weight Loss

When it comes to weight-loss success, Dr. Hill knows whereof he speaks. He's the cofounder of the National Weight Control Registry, a database of lifestyle information about more than three thousand people who have kept off an average of 67 pounds for six years. Almost every one of those folks engages in regular physical activity—and for most of them, it's walking.

"If I could change one thing in America to improve everyone's health, it would be to get people walking more," says Dr. Hill. And the most reliable way to walk more, he adds, is using a pedometer. A fascinating scientific study helps prove his point.

Ten Thousand Steps vs. Thirty Minutes

The study was conducted at the University of Tennessee by a team of three researchers, including Dixie Thompson, PhD, professor of Exercise, Sports, and Leisure Studies and director of the Center for Physical Activity and Health.

Dr. Thompson and her colleagues studied fifty-eight nonexercising women, with an average age of forty-five. They divided them into two groups. One group was told to take a brisk, thirty-minute walk on most (and preferably all) days of the week. (That's the same recommendation for daily exercise of any kind made by the surgeon general.) One group was told to walk 10,000 steps a day (a common recommendation for health and fitness made by pedometer experts—later in this chapter, we'll look more closely at the whys and wherefores of that number).

Both groups wore "sealed" pedometers they couldn't read; later, the researchers used these to tally their amount of walking. The 10,000-a-day group wore a second, unsealed pedometer to monitor (and hopefully reach) their daily step goal. Now here's the fascinating part . . .

The group told to walk thirty minutes a day walked an average of 8,270 steps a day. The group told to walk 10,000 steps a day walked an average of 10,159 steps a day. In other words:

When researchers told people who weren't exercising to either take a brisk thirty-minute walk a day or walk 10,000 pedometer-counted steps a day, the people who used the pedometer walked an average of <u>a mile more a day</u> (2,000 steps).

It's not that the women who were told to walk thirty minutes didn't walk at all—on the days they took a walk, they typically reached 10,000 steps. But on the days they didn't walk, they were relatively inactive. In contrast, the 10,000-steps-a-day group was active on *most days*—and therefore more active overall. "The 10,000-step approach gets people more active every single day," Dr. Thompson told us.

And let's look at those results from the surgeon general's point of view: the women who wore a pedometer and tried to achieve 10,000 steps of walking a day *met* the surgeon general's recommendation for a healthy dose of daily activity; the women who tried to take a thirty-minute walk every day *didn't* meet it.

"It is incredible that the pedometer could help sedentary people meet the criteria for the surgeon general's recommendation, because that goal is so rarely achieved," says Caroline Richardson, MD—an assistant professor in the Department of Family Medicine at the University of Michigan, a research scientist at the VA Medical Center in Ann Arbor, and an expert in using pedometers to help people walk more.

How can a diminutive device you clip to your waist transform you from a couch potato to a happy recruit in the surgeon general's activity army?

THE PERSUASIVE PEDOMETER

A pedometer, Dr. Richardson told us, helps you do what behavioral scientists say you must do to make any positive change: set a goal; monitor it yourself; and feel the satisfaction of success once you've reached it. With a pedometer as your sidekick, you can . . .

Set a Concrete, Reachable Goal

To set and reach any goal, you have to know two things: *where you're at right now,* and *where you want to go.* "In the science of behavior change and motivation, the 'theory of self-regulation' says that you can't change your behavior if you don't know what your behavior is," explains Dr. Richardson. "If you don't know how many steps you're taking, for example, you can't increase your steps. And nobody knows how many steps they're taking without a pedometer—in fact, they're usually way off."

Bottom line: pedometers allow you to know how much you're walking—and then set a goal to walk more.

Get Instant Feedback

Once you've set your goal, the pedometer tells you whether or not you're reaching it—instantly.

"Pedometers give you instantaneous feedback," says Dr. Hill. "If my goal is 11,000 steps a day, I can look at my pedometer and know—right away—how I'm doing that day. And that's why it's so powerful—if you can periodically check in to see how you're doing, you're much more likely to achieve your goal."

Compared to a pedometer, other kinds of feedback don't make the grade. "If I'm trying to walk thirty minutes a day, what do I do for feed-back?" asks Dr. Hill. "Start a stopwatch every time I get up and walk around? That's not going to work. Pedometers provide a simple and instant way to track progress."

Make the Small Changes That Drive Success

The best way to use a pedometer is to first figure out the number of steps you typically walk each day and then increase that number—*in small amounts.*

"Small changes drive success," says Dr. Hill. He didn't always think that way. But now he knows better.

"I spent most of my career trying to get people to make *big* lifestyle changes," he told us. "They made them—but they didn't stick with them. I've done a total about-face in my approach to lifestyle change because now I understand that *small changes* are what work."

How does a pedometer fit into that philosophy? "Let me give you an example," he says. "A patient of mine decides to follow the physical activity recommendations that accompany the dietary guidelines from the USDA: to get anywhere from thirty to ninety minutes of moderate to intense phys-ical activity on most days of the week. Well, if he's like many of the over-weight people I work with, he probably hasn't been off a couch in six months. Even thirty minutes of physical activity isn't going to be easy for him. But he's determined to give it a try. He joins a gym, works out a couple of days a week for two to three weeks—and then stops. *Why* did he stop? Because the change was too big to sustain. But with a pedometer, he doesn't have to achieve a big goal right away, like exercising for thirty minutes most days of the week. Instead, he determines how many steps he takes each day, and then he increases that number by a *little bit.* He moves *toward* his goal, little by little."

Small changes allow you to get motivated and stay motivated—"until you've made a big, extraordinary change," says Dr. Hill. And when you've achieved a big change through a series of small changes, it's much more likely you'll *stay* changed.

Feel Good About Yourself

Another important part of increasing your level of physical activity is what behavioral scientists call *self-efficacy*, says Dr. Richardson: you have to *believe* you can reach the goal. With a pedometer, that's easy. She gives an example:

"I tell one of my patients to increase her steps by 1,000 a day. She walks down the hall and back and sees that she's just put 100 steps on her pedometer. She says to herself, 'Wow, I just got 100 steps—I'm going to walk down that hall again.' "

That feel-good experience is quite different from what typically happens when a well-meaning doctor tells you to "get more exercise."

"When you're sedentary and a physician tells you to exercise more, you really don't know where to start," says Dr. Richardson. You might work out too hard and feel lousy afterwards, she points out. You might *still* feel like a failure, because you really don't know if you exercised enough. But with a pedometer, you have a concrete goal. You know exactly what you need to do and whether you've done it or not. And when you do it, you feel good about yourself.

YOUR PEDOMETER PROGRAM

You're ready to put on a pedometer and see where it takes you. But you quickly discover there are hundreds of pedometers on the market, some selling for as little as a dollar. How do you choose?

Accuracy is the most important feature. You don't want a pedometer that undercounts (so you never reach your goal) or overcounts (so you think you've reached it but haven't). Here's how to get the most accurate pedometer without paying a leg and a leg.

Buy an Accurate Device

"There is controversy among scientists as to which pedometers are the most accurate," says Dr. Thompson. She should know. Researchers in her department at the University of Tennessee tested thirteen different pedometers for accuracy, from the Accusplit Alliance to the Yamax Digi-Walker.

They designated one pedometer as the "gold standard" for accuracy, based on previous studies, and compared it to the others. Five of the pedometers "significantly overestimated steps" (by as much as 45 percent), while another five "significantly underestimated" them (by up to 25 percent). What's a would-be walker to do?

Spend more than five dollars. "You get what you pay for," says Dr. Thompson. She recommends staying away from cheaper pedometers (there are a lot of them out there), choosing one in the $20 to $25 price range. Dr. Hill offers similar advice.

Base your choice on price, he told us. There are basically three price levels for pedometers, he says. "Those under $5 are often toys. Those in the $5–$15 range are decent, but may not be completely accurate. And those ranging from $15 to $20 and higher are very accurate." (Though even the best pedometers are getting less and less expensive, he notes.)

Buy a pedometer you can return. When you get your pedometer home, put it on, set it, and take 100 steps—while also counting the steps yourself. If the pedometer is more than 5 percent inaccurate—if the display shows fewer than 95 steps or more than 105—return it, says Dr. Thompson.

If you're overweight, choose a "piezoelectric" rather than a "spring-levered" pedometer. There are two basic types of pedometers. The *spring-levered* variety has a spring and a lever arm that moves with each step, hitting a contact point that registers the step. The *piezoelectric* variety (also called an *accelerometer*) contains a "strain gauge"—a tiny device that detects move-

PEDOMETER.COM: USING THE WORLDWIDE WEB TO WALK MORE

Wait a worldwide second! Isn't sedentary surfing the very opposite of a more active lifestyle? Not necessarily, says Dr. Caroline Richardson, who's an expert in helping people walk more by uploading information from a pedometer to an Internet site.

"In the future, most people will have enhanced pedometers that upload information to the Internet," she told us. But why would anyone want to do that? Doesn't it make the simple process of counting and increasing steps a whole lot more complicated?

"It has so many advantages," says Dr. Richardson. And a tour of one of the current sites—www.fitbug.net—shows just what those advantages are. Once you've bought their pedometer and signed up with their program, you can see graphs of your daily steps . . . receive e-mails from a "personal walking coach," encouraging you to walk more or congratulating you on a job well done . . . join a "football league" (or set one up with your friends, family, or coworkers) that allows you to have weekly step competitions. The site also times, tracks, and tallies (in attractive graphs) other lifestyle information (like calorie intake and weight), all with the goal of encouraging and motivating you to keep walking for better health and a trimmer body.

Dr. Richardson also envisions a day in which the logic of preventive medicine (using lifestyle interventions to delay or stop a disease rather than spending thousands of dollars to treat it) will emerge as the new paradigm in health care. In that scenario, she says, physicians will prescribe pedometers. And the government will actually pay people to walk—for example, a person with blood sugar problems, to help stop type 2 diabetes. Super-accurate, downloadable pedometer data (where patterns of cheating are easy to detect) will prove whether or not those patients are putting in their steps and should be paid.

ment. It's so accurate that it can tell the difference between a step and a jiggle (like when you're riding in a golf cart or bus). "Piezoelectric pedometers are more accurate, particularly for people who are overweight," says Dr. Richardson.

Researchers at Cornell University compared the accuracy of piezoelectric and spring-loaded pedometers in overweight and obese people with a high BMI (body mass index, a measure of fatness) and large waist size. The spring-loaded pedometer was less accurate than the piezoelectric pedometer—and the higher the person's BMI and waist size, the more inaccurate it became. Why?

To function accurately, a spring-loaded pedometer must be vertical: straight up and down. A big belly makes a tilt quite likely. But tilt is not a factor with a piezoelectric pedometer.

Researcher recommendations. Dr. Thompson favors the New Lifestyles (piezoelectric) and Digi-Walker (spring-loaded) brands. "We have good success with these pedometers," she says. "They tend to count accurately and they tend to last." (Dr. Preuss is also a fan of the Digi-Walker—it's the pedometer he's been using for the past eight years.)

Dr. Richardson recommends any one of three pedometers: the Digi-Walker SMV 200, the Omron HJ 112 (piezoelectric), and the SportBrain.

"The Digi-Walker is very simple and very reliable," she says. "The Omron is not quite as user-friendly—it has four buttons instead of one, you have to play with it a bit to figure it out, and it's a little bit bigger. But it's got a lot of features people enjoy, like a clock that automatically resets the step counter to zero at midnight. The SportBrain isn't the best or most accurate pedometer, but you can upload your steps onto a Web site and get detailed data that is amazing."

Wear It Where It Works

For best results, wear the pedometer on your waistband or belt, two to six inches on either side of your belly button, says Dr. Hill. What about a dress without a waistband or belt? "Try wearing the pedometer on your undergarment," he advises.

If you're overweight, wear the pedometer on the side of your hip, where your arm hangs by your side.

Figure Out Your Current Daily Steps—
And Then Add More

You've bought a pedometer . . . tested it for accuracy . . . and clipped it to your waist. Now what? Don't do anything else differently—at least for a couple of days . . .

Option 1: Add 2,000 steps—and then individualize. "Wear your new pedometer for three to seven days," says Dr. Hill. At the end of each of those days, write down the number of steps your pedometer has recorded—2,009, 3,471, 4,682, whatever. After three to seven days, calculate the average, dividing the total number of steps by the total number of days. (For example: 21,000 steps divided by seven days equals 3,000 steps a day.) You have determined your baseline—your average daily number of steps.

"For the next week, increase your baseline by 2,000," says Dr. Hill. In other words, if your baseline was 6,000, you'd be walking 8,000 steps a day. (And in a moment, we'll suggest some fun ways to get those "extra" steps.) Why 2,000?

It's about one mile, or fifteen to twenty minutes of additional walking per day—an increase just about anybody can do, he says. (*Small changes drive success . . . small changes drive success . . .*)

Many experts think you should continue to increase your weekly total, week by week, until you reach 10,000 steps a day, a number widely considered ideal for weight maintenance. Dr. Hill disagrees—for a couple of different reasons.

"Once people add 2,000 steps to their daily average, they don't stop," he says. "They get it. They say to themselves, 'Oh, if I could do 2,000, maybe I could do more.' And they do."

Also, he says, a goal of 10,000 is too big and too far off—a large and potentially discouraging change.

Finally, a person's daily step count should reflect his or her lifestyle, not an arbitrary number. For some, 10,000 may not be enough. For others, 8,000 may be optimal for health.

"I believe people should achieve what they can as individuals, getting in as many steps as possible, given their health and lifestyle," says Dr. Hill.

Option 2: Add 1,200 steps a day each week—until you reach 10,000. Dr. Richardson favors a slightly different approach.

"Wear a pedometer for seven days to determine your baseline," she advises. Then add 1,200 steps per day, for the first week. "That's enough steps to be a bit challenging, but not so many that it's impossible," she says. Add an additional 1,200 the second week. And 1,200 more the third. And 1,200 more the fourth. Etcetera, until you reach 10,000.

But, like Dr. Hill, she counsels you to individualize the amount, depending on your situation. "With my patients, I constantly adjust the 1,200-per-day number and the overall number, depending on what the person can do. If he's not making his goal, or making only half his goal, I don't add 1,200 steps a week."

However, she thinks 10,000 steps a day is a good goal for most people—*because* it's not easy to achieve. "It's a challenge to reach 10,000 steps," she says. "You have to go on almost an hour walk per day, or do a lot of little walks throughout the day. So if you're trying to maintain your weight, 10,000 isn't good enough—it's *excellent.*" And that kind of difficult-to-achieve goal is the goal you're *most* likely to reach, she says.

"Thousands of studies on goal setting show that *high, hard goals* are what maximize success—and it doesn't matter how high or hard they are, as long as the person thinks there is a reasonable chance of achieving the goal," says Dr. Richardson. "People *like* high, hard goals—they're motivating and fun. Adding 1,200 steps per week, with a 10,000 goal, is a high, hard goal that almost anybody can reach if they try. If it's too high, the person can adjust."

A Word of Caution

However many steps you decide to take per week, if you have *any* question about your capacity to walk more (because, for example, you have diabetes or are very overweight or have another physical problem), Dr. Preuss counsels you to see your physician before you begin. "Your doctor may want to modify the number of steps you're planning to take," he says.

Find Little Ways to Do a Lot More

How do you increase your steps? An obvious way is to go for a daily walk of twenty or thirty minutes, or more. But that's not the only way.

Ten smart strategies. Researchers in the Department of Sports Medicine at the University of Southern Maine studied thirty-four people involved in an eight-week "pedometer-based lifestyle intervention." They found people typically chose one or more of ten strategies to increase their daily steps. They walked:

- to a meeting or on a work-related errand

- after work

- before work

- at lunch

- on the weekend

- while traveling

- with the dog

- to a destination, like work or a store

- after parking farther away from a destination

- using the stairs rather than the elevator

In *The Step Diet*, Dr. Hill offers many creative ways to increase daily steps at work, when out and about, and at home with family and friends. They include:

Work: Take two ten-minute walks during the day; walk to a rest room, soda machine, or copy machine on a different floor; walk a few laps around your floor during breaks; take five-minute walking breaks from your computer; get off the bus earlier and walk the extra blocks to work; walk while using a speaker or cordless phone; find a lunch spot that is at least a ten-minute walk each way.

Out and about: Return your grocery cart to the designated storage area; walk at the airport while waiting for your plane; take several trips to unload your groceries from your car; avoid drive-throughs—get out of your car and walk inside; walk around the local flea market or mall; walk to your nearest mailbox to mail a letter instead of leaving it for the mail carrier to pick up; walk around the field or the gym at your kids' games; pick up litter in your neighborhood or park.

At home with family and friends: Instead of reading the newspaper or watching the news on TV, put on your Walkman and listen to the news while you take a walk; walk around the living room during TV commercials (close to 1,000 steps during a one-hour program!); occasionally walk to the TV to change the channel; go up and down the stairs with laundry or other household items separately instead of combining trips; empty wastebaskets every day; walk to a neighbor's or friend's house instead of phoning; rake the leaves in your neighbor's yard.

Stick with It

Well, all of that *sounds* good. But you've been there and done that—and then stopped doing that. (Maybe your basement is a museum of good intentions, with a NordicTrack, AbMat, and Bowflex side by side in the Hall of Dashed Hopes.)

"There's a six-month, 50 percent dropout rate for most physical activity programs, and that's probably true for pedometers as well," says Dr. Richardson. But there's a way to improve those odds . . .

Find some pedometer pals. "If you give a person a pedometer and tell her to walk 10,000 steps a day, but nobody knows she has a pedometer, and she doesn't know anybody with a pedometer—chances are good that she'll throw the thing in a drawer after a week and never look at it again," says Dr. Richardson. But if you give everybody in her office a pedometer . . . and there's a chart on the wall tracking each person's progress . . . and every day people are comparing their step counts . . . and planning a walk at lunch—chances are very good that in a year she'll *still* be using the pedometer.

"Social support and group activity has an effect on any kind of physical activity, and it seems to make a huge difference with pedometer-based walking," says Dr. Richardson. (And may be more important for women than for men, she adds.)

So count your steps—but also count on family members, friends, or coworkers to help you do it.

Take a 3,000-mile walk. Put up a map of America and decide to walk across it, tracking your progress day by day, says Dr. Richardson. You can find "challenge charts" to help you track huge distances at www.the pedometercompany.com.

Walk and don't worry. "When it comes to pedometers, we've found there are three different types of people," says Dr. Hill. "For some people, a pedometer seems like the answer to their prayers. You give them a pedometer and they say, 'Oh my god, I've been looking for this all my life.' They use it and they wouldn't be caught without it."

STRENGTH TRAINING: GIVE FAT LOSS A LIFT

"On average, women in the middle years of their lives gain one to two pounds a year, and most of this is assumed to be fat," says Kathryn Schmitz, PhD, an assistant professor in the Center for Clinical Epidemiology and Biostatistics at the University of Pennsylvania, in Philadelphia. (Our observation is that men aren't doing much better.) Could exercise help stop the gain?

To find out, Dr. Schmitz studied 164 overweight or obese women, aged twenty-five to forty-four. Half the women were asked to do *strength training* (lifting weights) twice a week for two years. They had four months of lessons and supervision, and ongoing support from skilled fitness coaches. Each session lasted about one hour, and about 70 percent of the women stuck with the program.

The other half were given a brochure recommending thirty minutes of vigorous exercise on most days of the week. Both groups were told not to change their diets.

Dr. Schmitz reported the results of her research at the American Heart Association's annual conference in 2006:

Four percent less total fat. Those lifting weights had a decrease in total body fat of almost 4 percent. Total body fat stayed the same in the other group.

Fourteen percent less belly fat. Over the two years of the study, both groups had an increase in deep belly fat (the so-called *visceral fat* linked to in-

---

There's another group that doesn't take to pedometers, he says. They try it and don't like it, for whatever reason.

But there's a third group, says Dr. Hill. And until recently he didn't know they were out there. "These people put on a pedometer, see how sedentary they are, and start walking regularly—*without* the pedometer. All they needed was a wake-up call."

Which means, he says, that everybody who quits using a pedometer isn't a fitness failure—as long as they keep walking.

Keep walking—that's the perfect motto for this chapter. Keep walking. And keep your extra weight off for good.

creased risk for heart disease and type 2 diabetes). But those lifting weights had a *seven* percent increase, while those who didn't had an increase of *twenty-one* percent.

"What we've been able to show is that women ages twenty-five to forty-five who do twice-weekly strength training limited the increases in their deep belly fat over a two-year period," said Dr. Schmitz. And strength training had benefits beyond fat busting. "It was really empowering to these women," said Dr. Schmitz. "It made them feel like they were more capable in the rest of their lives."

Dr. Schmitz also recommends strength training for the over-sixty-five set: "Some of what we considered to be the inevitable frailty of advanced aging is, in fact, not inevitable, and may be preventable and even reversible with strength training."

The routine used in the study consisted of strength-training exercises for all major muscle groups, including chest, upper back, lower back, shoulders, arms, buttocks, and thighs. But don't go out and start weightlifting on your own—you might hurt yourself, says Dr. Schmitz. If you want to strength train, your best approach is the one used in her study: join a gym; find a competent instructor; learn how to do the exercises right; and have ongoing supervision that helps you safely increase the amount of weight you lift as you get stronger. If cost is prohibitive, says Dr. Schmitz, see if your insurance might pay for a gym membership, or ask about the YMCA/YWCA scholarship programs for discounted memberships.

PEDOMETER RX

Many scientific studies show that walking with a pedometer can help you lose fat. But a pedometer can also help you get healthier in all kinds of *other* ways.

Lower blood sugar levels. Eighteen women with a family history of type 2 diabetes were given pedometers and a goal of walking 10,000 steps a day. After eight weeks, their average number of steps per day increased from 4,972 to 9,213 (an 85 percent increase)—and their blood sugar was significantly lower (*Preventive Medicine*, 2003).

Healthier heart patients. Heart patients who used pedometers for six months had better scores in tests of "functional status" (distance walked in six minutes, and lung capacity) than heart patients who didn't use them (*Journal of Cardiac Failure*, 2005).

Arthritis relief. Thirty-four men and women with osteoarthritis of the knee were enrolled in either an arthritis self-management program or that program *and* instruction in the use of a pedometer, with the goal of increasing daily step count by 30 percent. At the end of six months, the pedometer group was walking 23 percent more per day—while the nonpedometer group was walking 15 percent less. The pedometer group was also walking more easily and faster. And they had a 21 percent gain in leg strength, compared to a 3.5 percent loss in the nonpedometer group (*Journal of the American Geriatric Society*, 2003).

Lower cholesterol. Twenty-seven menopausal women aged forty to sixty were divided into two groups: one didn't exercise and the other walked with a pedometer. The pedometer group walked an average of about 2,000 more steps per day—and had greater decreases in total cholesterol. The more daily steps they took, the lower their cholesterol (*BMC Women's Health*, 2002).

Lower blood pressure. Thirty-two men (average age forty-seven) with high blood pressure were instructed to walk 10,000 or more steps a day. Among those who walked 13,000 or more steps a day, average blood pressure fell from 149/99 to 139/90 (*Hypertensive Research*, 2000).

Living better with lung disease. Twenty-one patients with serious lung disease (chronic obstructive pulmonary disease) were given typical rehabilitation or rehabilitation and counseling in how to use a pedometer. The pedometer group walked 1,430 more steps a day after receiving the pedometer. "The use of the pedometer," concluded the researchers, "is a feasible addition to pulmonary rehabilitation which may improve outcome and maintenance of rehabilitation results" (*Patient Education and Counseling*, 2006).

Resource Guide

If you want to order and/or learn more about the nutritional supplements and herbs discussed and recommended in *The Natural Fat-Loss Pharmacy*, there are many commercial and informational resources you can consult. In addition, many resources provide information about, and allow you to participate in, effective weight-loss and fitness programs. On the following pages, you'll find lists of some of these resources, organized into four sections.

Section I: In this section you'll find general resources for obtaining the supplements and herbs discussed in *The Natural Fat-Loss Pharmacy*, at retail stores and on the Internet.

Section II: This section, which offers resources for each of the supplements and products recommended in *The Natural Fat-Loss Pharmacy*, is organized by chapter, and it includes books for more information and Web sites for obtaining products. As throughout the Resource Guide, the books are organized by date of publication, and the Web sites are listed alphabetically.

Section III: Here you'll find resources for credible weight-loss programs. *The Natural Fat-Loss Pharmacy* presents an effective dietary approach to weight loss in Chapter 13, *Easy Calorie Control*. But you may prefer to explore other weight-loss programs. Section III gives you a list of books and Web sites where you can find out more about such programs.

Section IV: This section lists resources for fitness programs. There is an effective, pedometer-based activity program in Chapter 14,

Step Right Up to Weight Control, but you may favor another type of fitness program, and we want to give you as many choices as possible. This section provides a list of books and Web sites about fitness.

Section I

The following list includes general resources where you can purchase the supplements and herbs discussed in *The Natural Fat-Loss Pharmacy.* You will find Web sites and retail stores (drugstores, supermarkets, superstores, and supplement and natural product stores). Many Web sites offer print catalogs and provide ordering by phone. Many retail stores maintain Web sites. This is a partial listing of well-established Web sites and retail stores (listed alphabetically, and not in order of preference) that sell multiple brands of nutritional supplements and herbs.

Web Sites

www.drugstore.com

www.shopping.com

www.swansonvitamins.com

www.vitacost.com

www.vitaminlife.com

www.vitaminshoppe.com

www.vitaminworld.com

Drugstores, Supermarkets, Superstores, and Supplement and Natural Product Stores (National Chains)

Albertsons

Costco

CVS

Duane Reade

Eckerd

Family Pharmacy

GNC

Kroger

Longs Drug Stores

Rite Aid Pharmacy

Safeway

Target

Trader Joe's

Vitamin Shoppe

Vitamin World

Walgreens

Wal-Mart

Whole Foods Market

Wild Oats

Section II

This section includes informational and commercial resources for each of the supplements and products recommended in *The Natural Fat-Loss Pharmacy.* The section is organized by book chapter.

CHAPTER 1: SIP YOUR FAT AWAY

Books

Lose Weight with Green Tea: A Safe Weight-Loss Method That Works by Patricia Rouner (Smith House Press, 2005).

The Green Tea Lifestyle: One Couple's Discovery of Healthy Weight Loss Without Dieting by Keith and Gillian Bales (Trafford Publishing, 2004).

The Green Tea User's Manual by Helen Gustafson (Clarkson Potter, 2001).

Green Tea for Health and Vitality: Healthful Alternative Series by Jorg Zittlau (Sterling, 1999).

All About Green Tea by Victoria Dolby, MPH (Avery, 1998).

The Book of Green Tea by Diana Rosen (Storey Publishing, LLC, 1998).

Green Tea: The Natural Secret for a Healthier Life by Nadine Taylor, MS, RD (Kensington, 1998).

The Green Tea Book: China's Fountain of Youth by Lester A. Mitscher, PhD, and Victoria Dolby (Avery, 1997).

Web Sites

Sources of information about green tea

www.greentealovers.com/greenteahealthdietweightloss.htm

www.itoen.com

www.japanesegreenteaonline.com/weightloss.htm

www.merutea.com

www.peets.com

www.republicoftea.com

Sources for ordering supplements recommended in the book

www.teavigo.com (informational Web site)

Teavigo

www.amazon.com

www.fubaohealthstore.com

www.herbspro.com

www.naturalnutrionals.com

www.organicpharmacy.org

www.vitacost.com

www.vitaminshoppe.com

www.wholehealthproducts.com

Schiff Green Tea Diet

www.amazon.com

www.doctorstrust.com

www.iherb.com

www.swansonvitamins.com

www.vitaminwarehouse.com

ThermoGreen Tea Caps (Universal Nutrition)

www.amazon.com/health

www.a-z-nutrition.com/thteaca.html

www.vitadigest.com/universal-green-tea.html

www.vitamaker.com/universal-green-tea.html

www.vitamindeal.com/universal-green-tea.html

www.wholesalesupplementstore.com

CHAPTER 2: LOSE BODY FAT—WITHOUT DIETING OR EXERCISE

Web Sites

Sources of information about CLA

www.wisc.edu/fri/clarefs.htm (a comprehensive database of references to scientific studies about CLA)

Sources for ordering products recommended in the book

www.tonalin.com (informational Web site)

Tonalin CLA

www.doctorstrust.com

www.drugstore.com

www.gnc.com

www.iherb.com

www.lifeextensionvitamins.com

www.puritan.com

www.sourcenaturalscatalog.com

www.swansonvitamins.com

www.thecatalog.com
www.vitabase.com
www.vitadigest.com
www.vitaminlife.com
www.vitaminshoppe.com
www.vitaminworld.com

CHAPTER 3: STOP YOUR BODY FROM MANUFACTURING EXTRA FAT

Web Sites
Sources of information about HCA
   www.supercitrimax-cs.com (informational Web site)
Sources for ordering products recommended in the book
   Super CitriMax Clinical Strength can be found in these products
      Diab-X, www.provenresultshealth.com
      Health Through Nutrition Recomposize, www.gohtn.net/
      productsWeight.asp
      Lean Balance, www.leanbalance.com
      Metabolife Green Tea Formula, www.metabolife.com
      Metabolife Ultra, www.metabolife.com
      Metabolife Ultra Caffeine Free, www.metabolife.com
      Royal BodyCare Bioshape, www.rbcinfo.com/bioshape.html
      SkinnyWater, www.skinnywater.com
      Smartburn, www.smart-burn.com
      Swanson Health Products, Super CitriMax Clinical Strength,
      www.swansonvitamins.com
      Vitamin World Super CitriMax Full Strength,
      www.vitaminworld.com
      YouthFlow Weight Loss Support, www.youthflow.com
   *HCA-SX with niacin-bound chromium (ChromeMate) can be found
   in Super CitriMax from Now, which is sold at these Web sites*
      www.allvitaminsplus.com
      www.herbspro.com/nowfoods.htm
      www.luckyvitamin.com
      www.thecatalog.com
      www.vitadigest.com
      www.youthflow.com

CHAPTER 4: THE FAT THAT KEEPS YOU THIN

Books

The Coconut Diet: The Secret Ingredient That Helps You Lose Weight While Eating Your Favorite Foods by Cherie Calbom and John Calbom (Time Warner, 2005).

Eat Fat, Look Thin: A Safe and Natural Way to Lose Weight Permanently, Second Edition by Bruce Fife, ND (Piccadilly Books, Ltd., 2005).

Eat Fat, Lose Fat: Lose Weight and Feel Great with Three Delicious, Science-Based Coconut Diets by Mary Enig, PhD, and Sally Fallon (Hudson Street Press, 2005).

Know Your Fats: The Complete Primer for Understanding the Nutrition of Fats, Oils, and Cholesterol by Mary G. Enig, PhD (Bethesda Press, 2000).

Fats That Heal, Fats That Kill: How Eating The Right Fats and Oils Improves Energy Level, Athletic Performance, Fat Loss, Cardiovascular Health, Immune Function, Longevity, and More by Udo Erasmus (Alive Books, 1993).

Web Sites

Sources for ordering products recommended in the book

Slim Smart oil

www.bmsresources.ca/main.php?module5detail&id513730

www.nfh.ca/pages/products_slimsmart_en.html

Trident SAP 3:2 fish oil

www.nfh.ca/pages/products_fishoil_en.html

Monolaurin

www.amazon.com

www.familypharmacy.net

www.vitaminshoppe.com

CHAPTER 5: SHINE UP YOUR MUSCLES AND PARE DOWN YOUR FAT

Books

The Metabolic Syndrome Program: How to Lose Weight, Beat Heart Disease, Stop Insulin Resistance and More by Karlene Karst, RD (Wiley, 2006).

The Sugar Solution: Your Symptoms Are Real—And Your Solution Is Here by The Editors of *Prevention* Magazine with Ann Fittante, MS, RD (Rodale, 2006).

Lifting Depression: The Chromium Connection by Malcolm Noell McLeod, MD (Basic Health Publications, 2005).

User's Guide to Chromium: Don't Be a Dummy: Become an Expert on What Chromium Can Do for Your Health by Melissa Diane Smith (Basic Health Publications, 2002).

Reversing Diabetes: Reduce or Even Eliminate Your Dependence on Insulin or Oral Drugs by Julian Whitaker, MD (Warner Books, 2001).

Syndrome X: The Complete Nutritional Program to Prevent and Reverse Insulin Resistance by Jack Challem; Burton Berkson, MD; and Melissa Diane Smith (Wiley, 2001).

The Diabetes Cure: A Natural Plan That Can Slow, Stop, Even Cure Type 2 Diabetes by Vern Cherewatenko, MD, and Paul Perry (HarperCollins, 2000).

Chromium Picolinate: Everything You Need to Know by Gary Evans, PhD (Avery Publishing Group, 1996).

The Chromium Program: In Six Weeks You Can Lose Weight, Reduce Fat, Lower Cholesterol, Build Muscle, and Increase Energy by Jeffrey A. Fisher, MD (HarperCollins, 1995).

The Chromium Diet, Supplement and Exercise Strategy by Betty Kamen (Nutrition Encounter, 1990).

Web Sites

Sources for ordering products recommended in the book

ChromeMate (niacin-bound chromium)

www.amazon.com/health
www.hammernutrition.com
www.herbspro.com
www.houseofnutrition.com
www.iherb.com
www.nutritiongeeks.com
www.sourcenaturalscatalog.com
www.swansonvitamins.com
www.thecatalog.com
www.vitaminlife.com
www.vitaminshoppe.com

Cinnamon capsules

www.amazon.com/health
www.amermed.com

www.iherb.com
www.puritan.com
www.vitaminshoppe.com
www.wonderlabs.com

CHAPTER 6: LOWER YOUR CARBS—WITHOUT A LOW-CARB DIET

Web Sites
Sources of information about carbohydrate inhibitors
   www.phase2info.com (informational Web site)

Sources for ordering products recommended in the book
(PRODUCTS CONTAINING PHASE 2)

Best Weight Control Formulas Phase 2 (Swanson)
   www.amazon.com/health
   www.swansonvitamins.com

Carb Blaster (Herbs of Gold)
   www.discountvitaminsexpress.com.au (Australian site)
   www.fremantlehealthfoods.com (Australian site)
   www.goodlifedirect.com.au (Australian site)
   www.vitahealth.com.sg/SG/hogcb.html (Asia Pacific site)
   www.vitaminking.com.au (Australian site)

Carb Cutter (Health and Nutrition Systems International)
   www.affordablesupplements.com
   www.amazon.com/health
   www.drugstore.com
   www.valusport.com
   www.wholesalesupplementstore.com

Simple Steps Carb-Down (FoodScience of Vermont)
   www.allvitaminsplus.com
   www.herbspro.com
   www.ihealthtree.com

Carb Erase (Fitness Labs)
   www.nutritionexpress.com

Carb Extractor (HealthSource Inc.)
   www.healthsourceinc.com

Carb Intercept and Carb Intercept Chewable (Natrol)
   www.amazon.com/health

www.betterlife.com

www.drugstore.com

www.ihealthtree.com

www.iherb.com

www.natrol.com

www.vitacost.com

www.vitaminshoppe.com

Carb Shredder (Vitamin Shoppe)

www.amazon.com/health

www.vitaminshoppe.com

CarbSpa (TrimSpa)

www.amazon.com/health

www.ihealthtree.com

www.mysupplementstore.net

www.vitamaker.com

www.wholesalesupplementstore.com

CarboTame (Jarrow)

www.amazon.com/health

www.betterlife.com

www.fubao.bigstep.com

www.iherb.com

www.totaldiscountvitamins.com

Phase 2 Carbohydrate Blocker (Source Naturals)

www.amazon.com/health

www.ihealthtree.com

www.iherb.com

www.sourcenaturalscatalog.com

www.vitacost.com

Maximum Strength Carb Eliminator (Baywood)

www.amazon.com/health

www.betterlife.com

www.herbspro.com

www.ihealthtree.com

www.iherb.com

www.nationalsupplementcenter.com

www.valusport.com

www.vitadigest.com

www.wholesalesupplementstore.com

Phase 2 (Healthy Origins)
www.amazon.com/health
www.betterlife.com
www.herbspro.com
www.ihealthtree.com

Phase 2 (Natural Balance)
www.amazon.com/health

Phase 2 (Nature's Harmony)
www.nutritionhouse.com

Phase 2 (Now)
www.amazon.com/health
www.betterlife.com
www.herbspro.com
www.ihealthtree.com
www.iherb.com

Starch Stopper (Diet World)
www.dietworld.com

Starch Stopper (Innovite)
www.feelgoodnatural.com (Canadian site)

TheraSlim (ProThera)
www.protherainc.com

Carb Phaser 1000 (Biochem)
www.vigorousliving.com
www.vitacost.com

Carb-Ease (AdvoCare)
www.advocare.com
www.bmfnutrition.com
www.nutritionalhope.com
www.purenhealthy.com

Carbo-Slim
www.clinco.co.uk (UK site)
www.healthsmart.com
www.naturalhealthcaretoday.co.uk (UK site)

CHAPTER 7: STOP FAT FROM GETTING TO YOU

Books

The Fiber35 Diet: Nature's Weight Loss Secret by Brenda Watson, CNC, and Leonard Smith, MD (Free Press, 2007).

The Dietary Fiber Weight Control Handbook by Roger A. Brumback, MD, and Mary H. Brumback, RPh (BookSurge Publishing, 2006).

The F-Factor Diet: Discover the Secret to Permanent Weight Loss by Tanya Zuckerbrot, MS, RD (Putnam Adult, 2006).

High Fibre Cooking: Eating for Health Series by Anne Sheasby (Lorenz Books, 2003).

The Fiber for Life Cookbook by Bryanna Clark Grogan (Book Publishing Company, 2002).

Dr. Tooshi's High Fiber Diet: A Revolutionary Diet That Will Help You to Lose Weight, Prevent Cancer, Heart Disease, Diabetes, and Digestive Disorders by Alan M. Tooshi, PhD (Writer's Showcase Press, 2000).

Fiber Facts: Get the Truth Concerning Dietary Fiber by Rita Elkins, MH (Woodland Publishing, 1999).

Dietary Fiber: Its Surprising Range of Therapeutic and Protective Health Benefits by Shirley S. Lorenzani, PhD (McGraw-Hill, 1998).

The Fat Blocker Diet: The Revolutionary Discovery That Lowers Cholesterol, Reduces Fat, and Controls Weight Naturally by Arnold Fox, MD, and Brenda Adderly, MHA (St. Martin's Press, 1998).

Dr. Anderson's High-Fiber Fitness Plan: Your Complete Guide to Healthy Living by James W. Anderson, MD, and Nancy J. Gustafson, MS, RD (University Press of Kentucky, 1994).

Web Sites

Sources of information about chitosan

www.liposan.com (informational Web site)

Sources for ordering products recommended in the book

Chitosan (Now)

www.allvitaminsplus.com

www.amazon.com/health

www.ihealthtree.com

www.luckyvitamin.com

www.myvitanet.com
www.nutritiongeeks.com
www.thecatalog.com
www.vitaminlife.com

Chitosan (Natural Balance)
www.amazon.com/health
www.iherb.com
www.vitaminshoppe.com

Chitosan (Neutraceuticals Science Institute)
www.gonsi.com
www.health.emailprice.com
www.vitacost.com

Chitosan LipoSan Ultra (Pure Encapsulations)
www.bayho.com
www.myvitanet.com
www.naturalhealthyconcepts.com
www.smartbomb.com
www.totaldiscountvitamins.com

LipoSan Ultra Chitosan (Swanson)
www.amazon.com/health
www.swansonvitamins.com

Mixed Fiber Supplements
These supplements are widely available.
Please see the Web sites in section I.

CHAPTER 8: NATURAL CONTROL FOR FOOD CRAVINGS

Books
5-HTP: The Natural Way to Overcome Depression, Obesity, and Insomnia by Michael Murray, ND (Bantam, 1999).
5-HTP: Nature's Serotonin Solution by Ray Sahelian, MD (Avery, 1998).
Secrets of 5-HTP: Nature's Newest Super Supplement by Winifred Conkling (St. Martin's Paperbacks, 1998).

Web Sites
Sources of information about 5-HTP
www.5htp.com (informational Web site by Michael Murray, ND)

Sources for ordering products recommended in the book

5-HTP (Natural Factors)
www.amazon.com/health
www.iherb.com
www.vitapal.com

5-HTP (Nature's Way)
www.amazon.com/health
www.ihealthtree.com
www.vitacost.com
www.vitaminshoppe.com

5-HTP (Now)
www.allvitaminsplus.com
www.amazon.com/health
www.ihealthtree.com
www.iherb.com
www.myvitanet.com
www.organicpharmacy.org
www.thecatalog.com
www.vitaminlife.com

5-HTP (Solaray)
www.amazon.com/health
www.smallplanethealth.com
www.smartbomb.com
www.vitaminlife.com
www.vitaminshoppe.com

CHAPTER 10: MAKE EXERCISE MORE EFFECTIVE

Web Sites

Sources for ordering products recommended in the book

HMB

EAS
www.a1supplements.com
www.allstarhealth.com
www.amazon.com/health
www.bodybuilding.com

www.global-supplements.com
www.supplementwarehouse.com
www.vitadigest.com

Sci Fit

www.affordablesupplements.com
www.amazon.com/health
www.bodybuilding.com
www.wholesalesupplementstore.com

Twinlab

www.allstarhealth.com
www.amazon.com/health
www.bodybuilding.com
www.supplementwarehouse.com

BCAA

Sci Fit

www.bodybuilding.com
www.nutritiongeeks.com
www.vitadigest.com
www.wholesalesupplementstore.com

Jarrow

www.gotbody.com
www.health.emailprice.com

Now

www.amazon.com/health
www.wholesalesupplementstore.com

NSI

www.health.emailprice.com
www.vitacost.com

Optimum Nutrition

www.amazon.com/health
www.bodybuilding.com
www.health.emailprice.com
www.nutritiondiscounters.com
www.vitacost.com
www.vitadigest.com
www.wholesalesupplementstore.com

Universal Nutrition
www.amazon.com/health
www.bodybuilding.com
www.gotbody.com
www.health.emailprice.com
www.netrition.com
www.vitadigest.com
www.wholesalesupplementstore.com

Section III

CHAPTER 13: EASY CALORIE CONTROL

Books

100 Days of Weight Loss: The Secret to Being Successful on Any Diet Plan by Linda Spangle, RN, MA (Thomas Nelson, 2007).

The Perricone Weight-Loss Diet: A Simple 3-Part Plan to Lose the Fat, the Wrinkles, and the Years by Nicholas Perricone, MD (Ballantine Books, 2007).

The Volumetrics Eating Plan: Techniques and Recipes for Feeling Full on Fewer Calories by Barbara Rolls, PhD (Harper Paperbacks, 2007).

The Best Life Diet by Bob Greene (Simon & Schuster, 2006).

You: On a Diet: The Owner's Manual for Waist Management by Michael F. Roizen, MD, and Mehmet C. Oz, MD (Free Press, 2006).

Body for Life for Women: A Woman's Plan for Physical and Mental Transformation by Pamela Peeke, MD, MPH (Rodale, 2005).

The Complete Book of Food Counts, 7th Edition by Corinne T. Netzer (Dell, 2005).

Dr. Shapiro's Picture Perfect Weight Loss: The Visual Program for Permanent Weight Loss by Howard Shapiro, MD (Rodale, 2003).

Fight Fat After Forty: How to Stop Being a Stress Eater and Lose Weight Fast by Pamela Peeke, MD, MPH (Piatkus Books, 2003).

The Diet Cure: The 8-Step Program to Rebalance Your Body Chemistry and End Food Cravings, Weight Problems, and Mood Swings—Now by Julia Ross, MA (Penguin, 2000).

The Pritikin Principle: The Calorie Density Solution by Robert Pritikin (Time-Life Books, 2000).

The Fat to Muscle Diet: The Revolutionary Diet Plan That Boosts Your Calorie-Burning Power by Victoria Zak; Cris Carlin, MS, RD; and Peter D. Vash, MD, MPH (Berkeley, 1988).

Web Sites

Sources of information about weight loss

www.100dayschallenge.com
www.caloriecontrol.org
www.calorielab.com
www.drpeeke.com
www.hamptonsdiet.com
www.mypyramid.gov (USDA personalized eating plans)
www.nwcr.ws (The National Weight Control Registry)
www.pritikin.com
www.southbeachdiet.com
www.thefatlosstimes.com (news and information blog for weight loss)
www.weightwatchers.com

Sources for ordering products recommended in the book

Omega-3 Oil (Nordic Naturals)

www.amazon.com/health
www.appleadayandbeyond.com
www.herbsforliving.com
www.iherb.com
www.luckyvitamin.com
www.naturalhealthshoppe.com
www.omega-direct.com
www.vitacost.com
www.vitadigest.com
www.vitaminshoppe.com

Section IV

CHAPTER 14: STEP RIGHT UP TO WEIGHT CONTROL

Books

10,000 Steps a Day to Your Optimal Weight: Walk Your Way to Better Health by Greg Isaacs (Bonus Books, 2006).

The Complete Guide to Walking for Health, Fitness, and Weight Loss: A 52-Week Plan for Increased Energy and a Longer, Healthier Life by Mark Fenton (The Lyons Press, 2001).

Manpo-Kei: The Art and Science of Step Counting: How to Be Naturally Active and Lose Weight by Catrine Tudor-Locke, PhD (Trafford Publishing, 2006).

Pedometer Walking: Stepping Your Way to Health, Weight Loss, and Fitness by Mark Fenton and David R. Bassett Jr (The Lyons Press, 2006).

Prevention's Firm Up in 3 Weeks: Trim and Tone Your Trouble Zones for Your Best Body Ever by Michele Stanten (Rodale, 2006).

Walking: The Ultimate Exercise for Optimum Health (Audio CD) by Andrew Weil, MD, and Mark Fenton (Sounds True, 2006).

Bob Greene's Total Body Makeover by Bob Greene (Simon & Schuster, 2005).

Walk Away the Pounds: The Breakthrough 6-Week Program That Helps You Burn Fat, Tone Muscle, and Feel Great Without Dieting by Leslie Sansone (Center Street, 2005).

The Step Diet: Count Steps, Not Calories, to Lose Weight and Keep It Off Forever by James O. Hill (Workman Publishing Company, 2004).

8 Minutes in the Morning: A Simple Way to Start Your Day That Burns Fat and Sheds the Pounds by Jorge Cruise (Rodale, 2003).

Curves: Permanent Results Without Permanent Dieting by Gary Heavin (Putnam, 2003).

Shrink Your Female Fat Zones: Lose Pounds and Inches—Fast! From Your Belly, Hips, Thighs, and More by Denise Austin (Rodale, 2003).

Body for Life: 12 Weeks to Mental and Physical Strength by Bill Phillips (HarperCollins, 1999).

Web Sites

Sources of information about fitness

www.acefitness.org
www.americaonthemove.org
www.curvesinformation.com
www.emedicinehealth.com
www.fitbug.net
www.fitday.com
www.fitness.com
www.mywalks.com
www.shapeup.org
www.tbfinc.com
www.thepedometercompany.com
www.thewalkingsite.com
www.walkaboutmag.com
www.walking.about.com

www.walkinghealthy.com
www.weightlossforall.com
www.weightlossforgood.co.uk
www.whi.org.uk

Sources for ordering pedometers recommended in the book

Accusplit Digi-Walker

www.accusplit.com
www.amazon.com/electronics
www.pedometer.com
www.pedometersusa.com

New Lifestyles

www.new-lifestyles.com

Omron HJ 112

www.bodytronics.com
www.drugstore.com
www.onlinefitness.com
www.vkrshop.com

SportBrain (includes Internet connectivity)

www.amazon.com/electronics
www.bodytronics.com
www.istepx.com
www.vkrshop.com

Index

Hot flashes, 5-HTP for, 183–84
Hunger. *See* Appetite; Appetite control
Hydroxycitric acid. *See* HCA
Hydroxy methylbutyrate. *See* HMB
Hyperinsulinemia, 115, 128, 129
Hypothalamus, functions of, 192, 193,
    194, 195
Hypothyroidism, best supplements for, <u>162</u>

I

Immune system, supplements
    strengthening, 40, 50, 51, 64,
    228–29
Infections
    fungal, EGCG and, 39
    monolaurin supplements and, <u>97</u>
Inflammation
    body fat and, <u>65</u>
    CLA reducing, 50, 51, 67
    omega-3 fatty acids reducing, 98,
    315–16
Insomnia, 78, 184
Insulin
    chromium and, 105, 111–12, <u>117</u>
    cinnamon mimicking, <u>117</u>
    fat gain and muscle loss from, 129–30
    function of, 105, 127–28
Insulin resistance
    aging and, 116, 118
    blocking conversion of L-tryptophan to
        serotonin, 170
    carb blockers for overcoming (*see* Carb
        blockers)
    chromium preventing, 114, 118
    cinnamon regulating, <u>117</u>
    CLA and, 59
    development of, 115–16, 128
    health effects of, 115, 128–30, 138–39
    incidence of, 104
    weight loss and, 118, 129
Insulin sensitivity, chromium improving,
    113
Interferon-induced depression, 181–82

K
Kola nut, caffeine in, <u>245</u>, 246

L
L-arabinose, 136–37, 138, 142, 263
LCTs (long-chain triglycerides), 88–89, 93,
    94, 95, 97, 98
LDL cholesterol. *See* Cholesterol
Leptin, 192, 193
Leukemia, EGCG and, 40–41
LipoSan Ultra, 156
Liver disease, BCAA for, 229–30
Long-chain triglycerides. *See* LCTs
Longevity, chromium for, 105
Lou Gehrig's disease, EGCG and, 41
Low-calorie-density foods, for weight loss,
    302–4, 305–7
Low-carbohydrate diet
    alternative to (*see* Carb blockers)
    problems with, 130–32
Low-fat diets, problems with, 87, 130
L-tryptophan
    for appetite control, 172
    deficiency of, in diabetics, 179, 180
    EMS linked to, 169–70, 184, 186
    5-HTP as alternative to, 170, 171
    serotonin formation and, 169, 170
Lunches, in meal plan, 279
    Artichoke Pizza, 284
    Artichoke Pizza "Again," 285
    BBQ Chicken Salad, 284
    Beans and Onion Spread on Whole
        Wheat Crackers, 280
    Beef Vegetable Soup, 286
    Black Bean Roll-Up, 282
    Chef Salad with Whole Wheat
        Croutons, 282
    Chicken Caesar, 280
    Chickpea Dip with Tortilla Chips, 281
    Chinese Chicken and Vegetable Stir-Fry,
        279–80
    Coleslaw with Apple and Walnuts,
        282

About the Authors

HARRY PREUSS, MD, MACN, CNS, is a professor of physiology, medicine, and pathology at Georgetown University Medical Center, and is the author of more than 350 medical papers. He is a former Established Investigator of the American Heart Association and a former fellow of the National Institutes of Health. He was elected ninth Master of the American College of Nutrition (MACN) and has served as president of that prestigious organization. In addition, he is a Certified Nutrition Specialist (CNS) and was the president of that certification board for seven years. He recently received the Ragus Award for best research paper published in the *Journal of the American College of Nutrition* in 2006. He lives in Fairfax Station, Virginia.

BILL GOTTLIEB is the former editor-in-chief of Rodale Books and *Prevention* Magazine Books, and the author of several wellness books, including *Alternative Cures* (1.6 million copies sold), *The Calcium Key*, and *The DERMAdoctor Skinstruction Manual.* His articles on health and healing have appeared in *Reader's Digest, Prevention, Self, Men's Health,* and many other national magazines. He lives in Middletown, California.